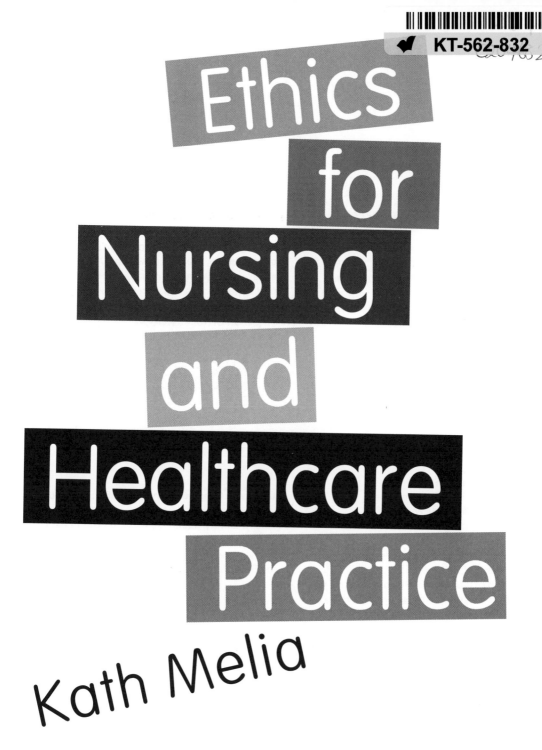

Ethics for Nursing and Healthcare Practice

Kath Melia

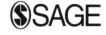

SAGE

Los Angeles | London | New Delhi
Singapore | Washington DC

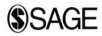

Los Angeles | London | New Delhi
Singapore | Washington DC

SAGE Publications Ltd
1 Oliver's Yard
55 City Road
London EC1Y 1SP

SAGE Publications Inc.
2455 Teller Road
Thousand Oaks, California 91320

SAGE Publications India Pvt Ltd
B 1/I 1 Mohan Cooperative Industrial Area
Mathura Road
New Delhi 110 044

SAGE Publications Asia-Pacific Pte Ltd
3 Church Street
#10-04 Samsung Hub
Singapore 049483

Editor: Alex Clabburn
Assistant editor: Emma Milman
Production editor: Katie Forsythe
Copyeditor: Solveig Gardner Servian
Proofreader: Neil Sentance
Marketing manager: Tamara Navaratnam
Cover design: Lisa Harper
Typeset by: C&M Digitals (P) Ltd, Chennai, India
Printed in Great Britain by Henry Ling Limited at
The Dorset Press, Dorchester, DT1 1HD

Library of Congress Control Number: 2013946251

British Library Cataloguing in Publication data

A catalogue record for this book is available from
the British Library

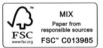

ISBN 978–0-85702–929–4
ISBN 978–0-85702–930–0 (pbk)

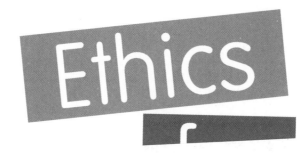

Ethics

This book is due for return on or before the last date shown below

2 4 MAR 2016		
2 6 MAY 2016		
2 7 MAY 2016		
1 9 JUN 2017		
2 0 JUL 2017		
1 7 DEC 2019		
10 / Feb / 2020		
3/8/21		

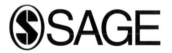

In memory of Neil MacCormick, Regius Professor of Public Law and the Law of Nature and Nations at the University of Edinburgh 1972–2008. Neil was a generous and inspiring colleague, whose work on practical reason in law and morality changed my view on the relationship between law and ethics and has influenced my thinking in writing this book. I hope that Neil would have approved of the result.

Contents

About the Author

Kath Melia, Professor of Nursing Studies at the University of Edinburgh, is a sociologist and health care researcher. A graduate of the Department of Social and Preventive Medicine, University of Manchester, she moved to Edinburgh to work in intensive care. Whilst working in the Nursing Research Unit at the University of Edinburgh on a study of ward organisation she completed a doctoral thesis on the occupational socialisation of nurses. She has a long-standing interest in the sociology of the professions and the nature of teamwork in the health care workforce. As an ESRC Research Fellow (2001–03) she studied the modernising of the NHS and its implications for the nursing profession as a managed occupation. Kath Melia has published in nursing and health care ethics.

Acknowledgements

First, my thanks to SAGE for the invitation to write this book; it has been an interesting task to bring sociology and law into what is essentially an ethics text. Thanks are due to colleagues at the National University of Singapore, who were generous with their ideas and time when, in 2009, I was fortunate to spend time as a Visiting Professor in the Centre for Biomedical Ethics to work on various projects, including the planning of this book. Especial thanks to Professor Alastair Campbell for the discussions we had, particularly those concerning the relationship between sociology and ethics. Also thanks to Dr Jacqueline Chin for many helpful discussions and for being a welcoming colleague with whom to share ideas and office space.

At SAGE I had the pleasure of working with Alison Poyner again; my thanks to her for her faith in the book from the outset and for her wise advice, particularly on the matter of explicitly including law and sociology in the book. To Susan Worsey, my thanks for her timely conversations and enthusiasm in the early stages of the work. Particular thanks to Emma Milman and Alex Clabburn for their editorial skill and relaxed approach to getting this book into production. Lastly, my thanks to Katie Forsythe for seeing the book through to press.

Once again, the Greek island of Symi has played its part in getting this work from the head to the page.

Kath Melia
Edinburgh, May 2013

Additional Online Material

This book is supported by an online resource with a number of free SAGE journal articles related to the book.

These papers are related to the main themes of the book and provide an opportunity to read beyond the discussion in the book. Some of the papers branch out a little further and discuss research (Gibson et al.; Suhonen et al.) and inter-professional teamwork (Ewashen). The further references included in these papers will provide further scope for following up the themes of the book.

Visit www.sagepub.co.uk/melia for free access to the following articles:

Begley, A. (2005) 'Practising virtue: a challenge to the view that a virtue centred approach to ethics lacks practical content', *Nursing Ethics*, 12(6): 622–37.

Cronqvist, A., Theorell, T., Burns, T. and Lützén, K. (2004) 'Caring about – caring for: moral obligations and work responsibilities in intensive care nursing', *Nursing Ethics*, 11(1): 63–76.

Denny, D.L. and Guido, G.W. (2012) 'Undertreatment of pain in older adults: An application of beneficence', *Nursing Ethics*, 19(6): 800–09.

Ewashen C. and McInnis-Perry, G. (2013) 'Inter professional collaboration-in-practice: the contested place of ethics', *Nursing Ethics*, 20(3): 325–35.

Gallagher, A. (2007) 'The respectful nurse', *Nursing Ethics*, 14(3): 360–71.

Gibson, S., Benson, O. and Brand, S.L. (2013) 'Talking about suicide confidentiality and anonymity in qualitative research', *Nursing Ethics*, 20(1): 18–29.

Hanssen, I. (2010) 'Utilitarian and common-sense morality discussions in intercultural nursing practice', *Nursing Ethics*, 17(2): 201–11.

Kangasniemi, M., Viitalahde K. and Porkka, S. (2010) 'A theoretical examination of the rights of nurses', *Nursing Ethics,* 17(5): 628.

Krishna, L. (2012) 'Best interests determination within the Singapore context', *Nursing Ethics*, 19(6): 787–99.

Krishna, L. (2011) 'Nasogastric feeding at the end of life: a virtue ethics approach', *Nursing Ethics*, 18(4): 485–94.

Schneider, D.G. and Ramos, F.R.S (2012) 'Moral deliberation and nursing ethics cases: elements of a methodological proposal', *Nursing Ethics*, 19(6): 764–76.

Izumi, S., Nagae, H., Sakurai, C. and Imamura, E. (2012) 'Defining end-of-life care from perspectives of nursing ethics', *Nursing Ethics*, 19(5): 608–18.

Snellman, I., Gedda, K.M. (2012) 'The value ground of nursing', *Nursing Ethics*, 19(6): 714–26.

Suhonen, R., Stolt, M., Veikko, L. and Leino-Kilpi, H. (2010) 'Research on ethics in nursing care for older people: A literature review', *Nursing Ethics*, 17(3): 337–52.

van Thiel, G. J. and van Delden, J. J. (2001) 'The principle of respect for autonomy in the care of nursing home residents', *Nursing Ethics*, 8(5): 419–31.

1
Introduction

Life is short, and Art long; the crisis fleeting, experience perilous, and decision difficult.

Hippocrates, 5th Century BC

Practical questions such as Should this patient continue to be fed artificially? are rarely simply technical matters. They carry concerns of fairness, rights, compromised freedom and justice. We often speak of the moral dimension of practice but it is perhaps more accurate to regard moral matters as being so bound up with the technical and social aspects of caring that to separate them out as a discrete item for discussion is not easy and possibly not helpful. The work of nurses and other health care professionals entails human contact. Decisions about care are matters of judgement; these are clinical judgements which, of course, also involve the patient. There will also be circumstances where this is not possible and the patient's relatives[1] and/ or legal representative can be involved. Nursing practice does not occur in a moral vacuum; the organisation of health care means that nurses work with other professionals making up the multidisciplinary team. The wider social context within which the decisions are made also has its influence on practice. Given all of this, we need to be clear about what ethics is and why we should be concerned with it in nursing practice.

Ethics, or moral philosophy, is the branch of philosophy that is concerned with the study of morals and the nature of morality. It is of practical value to clinicians in health care as it provides the language and concepts with which to argue for and justify a particular decision or action. In other words, it allows us to judge our own moral convictions and values against wider, socially accepted principles and rules for behaviour. Morality has to do with a sense of right and wrong. But where does this come from? Can it be taught?

---

[1] Throughout the book I use 'relatives' to refer to family and friends representing the patient's interests. I do so on the grounds that friends are related by friendship, whereas family need not imply friend.

This book concerns the moral dimension of nursing and health care practice. It is in no way a rule book, or even guide as to how to avoid ethical traps. Health care is a complex matter and nursing plays a central part in its practice. Situations arise in daily nursing practice which involve a decision to be made that is both a clinical and moral decision. In this book we take a down-to-earth, case-based approach to ethics. Essentially ethics is about the reasoning behind the decisions we take, and it forces us to think about what is the right thing to do in life. In the case of nursing practice, ethics is about how to decide how to act as a nurse.

In a society that has advanced to the point that a complex division of labour exists, health care is a professionalised activity and those being cared for will be, by and large, unknown to those doing the caring. Put simply, we have two sets of strangers, patients and professionals, who have to relate to each other in order to produce a working partnership, however transient. This is not, of course, to say that relationships do not develop; long-standing professional–patient relationships exist in all areas of practice. However, the point stands because even strong patient– professional relationships had to start somewhere. Nursing practice involves patient and professional coming together and arriving at a position where communication and care are brought about in a relationship which should be based on trust.

This book is an introduction to ethics for nursing and health care practice and stresses the importance of the social context in which this takes place. The idea is to introduce the moral philosophical language in which practical clinical issues[2] are discussed. The relationship between ethics and the law is a theme that runs through the book and so provides a basis for a good understanding of ethics and law as they relate to nursing practice. Ethical decisions are arrived at in practice in a social and legal context. Sociology is drawn upon where it can help to explain the social and organisational context of practice. Whilst this is an introductory text to ethics for practice, the aim is to discuss some of the complexities of ethical debate. The book starts from scratch, assuming no prior knowledge of ethics or law; however, the discussions can lead to a sophisticated level of debate, but a debate which remains firmly rooted in practice.

Ethics Morals and Practical Reasoning

Nursing practice is a complex business and it is expected, indeed assumed, that nurses will behave in an ethically acceptable way. In this book we explore exactly what this entails and through the discussion of cases we enter the world of the moral philosopher, and in so doing see what light moral philosophy can shed on the moral dimension of nursing. This book is not a comprehensive account of ethics for nursing

---

[2]'Issue' in this text carries the long-standing meaning and does not equate to 'problem'. Issue, meaning a topic for discussion, is a more neutral term used to describe matters worthy of discussion which may or may not be problematic. In many places I have used 'concerns' or 'matters' instead of 'issues' to avoid confusion for those who do equate 'issue' with 'problem'.

practice, rather it seeks to convey the central principles and their relationship to ethical debates in such a way as to nudge readers towards an examination of their own clinical experience and focus on the ethical aspects of practice.

Whilst ethics and morals have to do with right and wrong, they are not about dictating what we should and should not do. The distinction between morals and ethics is worth spending a little time on, although the terms are often used interchangeably. 'Morals' refers to the values and associated rules and practices by which people live, whereas 'ethics' is that branch of philosophy called moral philosophy, which is concerned with the study of morality.

Some writers prefer not to draw the distinction, pointing out that both words – ethics and morality – have their roots in words meaning 'customs' and as such are not really different, despite the distinction. 'Ethics' derives from the Greek *ethikos* which gives us the word 'ethos'. 'Morals' derives from the Latin *moralis*, meaning mores. Both words mean customs and ways of life followed and passed down through generations (Singer, 1994: 5). Singer also notes that ethics is a more neutral term and the word morality can convey a particularly religious resonance.

Within the health care literature I find that both ethics and morals are used interchangeably whilst at times the distinction is recognised, and so in this book I do not adopt a rigid approach to their use. Ethics is essentially about the study of morals and is generally about right and wrong. The terms ethics and morals whilst distinct can be used interchangeably without much harm coming to the discipline of moral philosophy. Nor, indeed, will any harm come to the study of ethics for nursing practice if we slip between the terms morals (the values and mores of behaviour) and ethics (moral philosophy, concerned with the study of morals).

The business of ethics is to examine the justifications offered for the various moral stances that people take on questions where there are various opinions and where decisions have to be made. In the face of an ethical dilemma where, by definition, it is not clear which action is the best option to take, moral philosophy offers the language and concepts with which to debate the matter. It also allows us to draw on a wider range of principles and theoretical positions which have stood the test of time and public debate. For example, the idea of respecting individual's rights to be treated in ways which are deemed to be acceptable and fair forms the basis of many discussions of resources. The use of resources can give rise to everyday questions which might appear to be trivial matters, such as making the best use of the available staff time on a shift in order to achieve the best outcomes for the patients on that unit.

A busy morning on a ward which has been the main admission ward overnight. There is a shortage of linen. There are not enough sheets to enable as many to be changed as would be desirable. The nurses on duty, having established that there will be no more sheets delivered to the ward until the afternoon, have to do the best they can. The

(Continued)

(Continued)

practical solution is to change those that cannot be left, and catch up later in the day with the rest when new stocks arrive.

There are organisational and maybe even financial considerations here. How should nurses react to this compromise of optimum patient care? In a busy ward the answer may be to make do and move on. But what if this is a common occurrence? If nurses always manage to cope, the situation may go unchanged, like the sheets! Is there an obligation to speak out in an attempt to make things better? And what if managing, quietly getting on with it, extends to other areas of care? Where should nurses hold, or even draw the line and speak out?

This question, which set out as a matter of what to do when there is a shortage of bed linen, has moral aspects to it. Moral choices, albeit small ones, are made in deciding who gets a clean sheet, and by default who does not. The right to a clean sheet is not an absolute one; our rights are often set against those of others – if one person's need is satisfied in a rationing situation, another person's is not. The greater need that one person has of the clean sheet does not alter the fact that the person with less need did not get a clean sheet. This not very dramatic example of moral choice is just one of many similar choices made by nurses in relation to the daily care of patients.

Ethical Debate

It is worth rehearsing the reasons why ethical debate is important; one of the main ones is that when vulnerable people are being cared for by strangers, there has to be an atmosphere of trust. We create this by developing a context for a professional– patient relationship. In order to achieve this we need some ground rules, and some of these rules are the concern of ethics. Ethical analysis and debate provide a way of examining and discussing the rights and wrongs of behaviour in health care. What is in the patient's best interests? How should we be caring for this patient? Is this a reasonable way to run a ward? How should we respond to aggressive behaviour in patients and their relatives? These are all questions for moral philosophy. We need a common language and a way of debating the rights and wrongs of how to go about nursing and health care, especially when things are not straightforward. We find this language in moral philosophy.

One of the interesting aspects of ethical debate is that there are no rights and wrongs about it. Leaving aside views that might be regarded as being beyond anyone's pale, ethical debate takes on board all moral arguments that are reasoned attempts at making a genuine effort to decide on the right action to take when faced with a difficult situation.

Philosophy is very much concerned with what is the right thing to do, how people justify their positions when making moral decisions. Moral decisions are very much like clinical decisions, they have practical connections and consequences and a social context. Ethics is a very practical business: decisions in health care have legal, moral, clinical, economic and psychosocial aspects.

In the midst of everyday practice there is rarely time to step back and ask are we doing the right thing, what should we do? In this day of protocols, evidence-based practice, audit trails and the rest, there is not a moral procedure book to consult. Yes, there are codes of conduct, ethical discussions, but in day-to-day practice there comes a point where practitioners working together with patients have to arrive at a decision; this is very much the social production of action. In other words, it is a practical matter, it is practical reasoning. Ethical debate gives an opportunity to explore moral issues using the language and concepts of moral philosophy. This means that we cannot take our usual ideas and stands on particular issues for granted, and this includes our prejudices. We do not tend to regard our own views and opinions on social matters as prejudices, they are just what we think. They may be strong enough convictions to make us disapprove of others who do not happen to share our opinion. When someone expresses what in our view is an unacceptable opinion during a general conversation, it can be difficult, especially if their assumption is that it is a shared view, and an unproblematic one at that. These views may be racist or sexist or offensive in some other way. These situations make two things clear: first, what we might assume to be a reasonable and common-sense view to hold is not necessarily a universal understanding; and second, it is not always easy to register our objection because it takes us out of the normal expectations and conventions of conversation in social life. Clearly there has to be a good deal of common understandings and beliefs if society is to function, and later in the book we return to this idea in a discussion of societal norms and expectations and the law.

My general point at this juncture is that we cannot always assume that others will automatically share the views that we, as individuals, hold about right and wrong. This is especially important for a professional group such as nursing where there is a need for shared values in the profession. There also has to be a means of engaging with a wide variety of patients who have other views and values.

In everyday life we do not normally try to investigate the justifications for the values that we hold. Moral philosophy at its simplest gives us a means by which to do this. As we have said, ethics is a deeply practical business; without real life practical examples to relate to, ethical debate is somewhat sterile. The discussions in this book are centred around a few classic and some hypothetical cases which give rise to ethical and sometimes legal and ethical debate. The clinical context can be supplied by the reader. The main aim of the book is to demonstrate, through discussion of some of the common themes of ethical debate, how such discussion can be of assistance in arriving at decisions in the practice of nursing and health care. The inclusion of classic and hypothetical cases giving rise to ethical and sometimes ethical and legal debate: this means that the book can be read and re-read at different stages in the reader's experience of practice.

In health care the patient is the prime concern. However, the social and clinical organisation of health care is complex and involves various health care professionals working in multidisciplinary teams, and often with the patient's relatives. The care takes place in a social context and so all concerned are constrained by social and economic circumstances, all of which makes the business of multi-disciplinary care often far from straightforward. The whole system operates on the basis of trust. Trust is a moral concept. We cannot see trust, it manifests itself through the behaviour of individuals towards one another. We have rules and regulations and laws, but these do not make the notion of trust redundant. Trust has to exist throughout the health care system from trust in the relationship which the patient has with the health care professionals to the inter-professional working relationships of the health care team which also require a basis of trust.

How Ought We to Live? From Aristotle (384–322 BC) to the 21st Century

Ethical questions that we raise today have a long history; the social context has changed, but the questions persist. In the spirit of giving the reader a good understanding of ethics I offer a preview, as it were, of Aristotle's approach to moral philosophy early in this book. We return to this in later chapters. It is useful to glimpse Aristotle's work early on in getting to grips with ethics because it is more relevant and engaging than one might be forgiven for thinking the ideas of a 4th-century BC Greek philosopher might be.

This question of how we ought to live is by no means new. The ancient Greek philosophers' central question was just that: how ought we to live? The goal for Aristotle was to grow towards the good. Their goal Singer (1994: 3) describes as 'wisdom about how to live our lives'. The idea of wisdom may seem rather arcane and not very 21st century, until we consider it in terms of judgement. Wise men, and wise women for that matter (although that term is too closely associated with witches to be entirely helpful), have existed through the ages. They have been looked to for help in times of difficult decision making. Believers will seek the wisdom of their gods in order to help when choices have to be made. If we move this idea of difficult choices from 4th-century BC into the 21st-century health care setting, we are talking about clinical judgement. Many clinical decisions taken in health care have a moral element and so we cannot escape the fact that clinical judgement and moral judgement are linked in practice.

Aristotle's work appears in many textbooks on medical ethics, biomedical ethics, and nursing ethics because Aristotle's work is practical, concerned as he was with questions about what constituted the good life and how one should live the good life. Campbell et al. (2005: 3) note that Plato in the 4th-century BC, in answering his own question 'What sort of person ought one to be?', said that the good person was guided by the 'form' of the good. Campbell et al. say that Plato was referring to

divine and eternal reality only imperfectly seen in everyday human existence, but supremely disclosed by the calm contemplations of wise men. (2005: 3)

Campbell et al. go on to note that we need to recognise that:

> great thoughts do not always mean good deeds, and that morality is essentially to
> do with our attitudes, behaviour and relations to one another. (2005: 3)

Some Christian writers, Aquinas being one, have according to Campbell (1984) added to Aristotle's theory the idea that the ideal way of being (of living) is consistent with God's design for humankind. In this way, Campbell explains, 'natural' and 'good' become fused. This is clear when we examine some of the ethical theories. Aristotle's response to Plato's 'What sort of person should we be?' question was pragmatic, according to Campbell et al., as:

> for Aristotle the qualities that make us human were shown in our thinking, our associations with each other and our functions as members of the natural order. (2005: 3)

Campbell et al. remind us that Aristotle and Hippocrates[3] approached their work in much the same way and

> began with observations of the actual world in which they lived, rather than beginning with theories about life, the universe and everything. (2005: 3)

This empirical approach – that is, starting with the 'facts' as observed – we will see was the approach taken by the 18th-century philosopher David Hume. It was, in his day, a break away from the more commonly encountered way of working when philosophers proceeded through reason and logic to theory. Campbell et al. describe this as the leap from Aristotle to Hume.[4]

Singer (1993: 88) reminds us that whilst in Western philosophy we look back to Greece and the great philosophers, Socrates, Plato and Aristotle, it was not the case that all their values are ones we would recognise today. There was no equality in society, slaves did not enjoy autonomy, newborns were not automatically preserved. We need, Singer cautions, to be careful not simply to adopt unthinkingly the ideas from the ancient Greek philosophers, because some would plainly not meet the expectations of contemporary life.

Singer tells us, for example:

> There was no respect for the lives of slaves or other 'barbarians'; and even among
> the Greeks and Romans themselves, infants had no automatic right to life. Greeks
> and Romans killed deformed or weak infants by exposing them to the elements

---

[3]Hippocrates, 5th-century BC Greek philosopher and teacher of medicine on the island of Kos. He is regarded as the 'father of medicine' and was author of the first code of practice for medicine, still read today in many medical schools at graduation ceremonies.

[4]Hume returns to this tale in Chapter 4.

> on a hilltop. Plato and Aristotle thought that the state should enforce the killing of deformed infants. (1993: 88)

We can see from this that the state has for centuries had a role in what we would now call 'health care ethics'. Also we can see most starkly in Singer's example that moral values can and do change. This is why there are no absolute rights and wrongs about moral debate.

One of the things that remains constant is human nature, a concern with doing the right thing with fairness and justice and working out the right thing to do, how to behave. Looking around the world this would seem something of a Utopian proposition with misuse of power, unnecessary wars, famines that could be ended if people behaved in a way that was decent. It is worth pondering for at least a few minutes what the world would look like if everyone behaved in the way that they are supposed to do. Police forces and armies would be redundant save for humanitarian work required as a result of natural disaster and accident. Fraud squads, anti-computer hacking teams, war correspondents, hours of medical and nursing staff time in Accident and Emergency departments could be saved and redeployed when drunks and related casualties are removed from the patient list. All very fanciful and, of course, dependent upon one vital definition of a condition that I slipped in at the start of this paragraph, namely what is the *right* thing to do? How does society arrive at an agreed version of the right thing to do?

Notwithstanding all this, Aristotle's work is particularly useful in relation to health care ethics because his work has resonance for today's practice. There is no need to read the original (equally no reason not to!). There are many introductions to Aristotle's work, and those writing in the field of bioethics make clear Aristotle's meanings when they draw upon his work. Aristotle's ideas have a very contemporary ring to them; the translations are to an extent responsible for this, and the style adopted makes it possible to draw a direct line from 4th-century BC ancient Greece to 21st-century Western health care ethics.

One of Aristotle's ideas that has utility in terms of ethics for nursing practice comes in his writing about habituation, in the sense of doing something repeatedly so that it becomes second nature – a habit. He says that 'moral virtues, like crafts, are acquired by practice and habituation' (Book II, 1103a14–b1). A virtue in the ancient Greek world was an excellence. Its meaning was not dissimilar from our notion of competence.[5] In an uncannily relevant example of prudence, or practical wisdom, Aristotle says:

> Prudence is not concerned with universals only; it must also take cognizance of particulars, because it is concerned with conduct, and conduct has its sphere in particular circumstances. That is why some people who do not possess [theoretical] knowledge are more effective in action (especially if they are experienced) than

---

[5]Competencies form the basis of the regulatory mechanisms used to approve university programmes in nursing. This is the case too with medicine and other health care professions.

others who do possess it. For example, suppose that someone knows that light flesh foods are digestible and wholesome, but does not know what kinds are light; he will be less likely to produce health than one who knows that chicken is wholesome. But prudence is practical, and therefore it must have both kinds of knowledge, or especially the latter. Here too, however, there must be some co-ordinating science. (Book VI, 1141b8–27)

Aristotle's discussion of nutrition nicely demonstrates the relevance of his thinking to today's health care, especially with his emphasis on practice. Indeed, Aristotle's view was that unless ethical theory was related to practical examples in life, it was poor philosophy. This is why the ethical debates we have in nursing move between theoretical, abstract principles and cases, clinical examples in everyday practice.

Working in the Theory–Practice Gap

Practice disciplines present particular challenges when it comes to the relevance of theoretical debate to the everyday practice. Moral philosophy can be rather abstract and theoretical, somewhat removed from the concerns of the practitioner faced with the need to make decisions and, importantly, the need to act. An under-staffed ward, where too many beds are currently occupied by patients who should have been either discharged home or transferred to a more appropriate unit, is not the place to have a theoretical discussion about justice and resources. Moral philosophy is characterised by a capacity to move between the theoretical ideas and practical examples.

In the nursing literature, and in that of other professionals in health care, there is much ink spilled over the matter of bridging the perceived gap between theory and practice. This idea on the first encounter appears to be a good one. However, on reflection not only does it prove to be of little help in seeing anything more clearly, but also the idea itself seems to be somewhat flawed. It is not clear what a bridge would look like and what it might link to. The same question might be raised in the case of a perceived gap between moral theory and nursing; that is, how do moral philosophy and ethical theory relate to everyday nursing practice?

> Eliciting informed consent from a patient who has mood swings, which make their capacity for taking decisions transient, is a practical matter. The patient's capacity for reason and decision making may change from day to day or even hour to hour.

This is the reality of daily care, a practical matter with theoretical underpinnings. This is not so much a gap to be bridged as a situation where different orders of knowledge and understandings are required. The practical and proper response at the time is important for good practice to result. This is not so much a theory–practice gap as a matter of there being a time and a place for these debates. A theoretical discussion of autonomy and the reasons why it should be respected can tell us why the principle of respect for autonomy is a good thing.

The gap is more one of perspective and changing priority depending on the situation; thus it is a gap between theory and practice. Working with or in this gap holds more promise than does bridging it. In a typical discussion of the theory–practice gap, the idea is that theory is 'all very well' until it is tried in practice, and it is then that the gap is encountered. This is not a purely nursing phenomenon: newcomers to any practice discipline will encounter experienced practitioners who may be more concerned with practicalities and appear to have little interest in theory. It may be that this is, in fact, the case. However, it is just as likely that experienced practitioners have adjusted to working with, or in, the gap and so know when it is appropriate to give more attention to the theory and when practical matters, albeit informed by theory, take precedence.

Making Judgements

Judgement is an essential clinical skill which comes with practice. However, the opportunity to have the discussion in a calmer setting is a useful way of considering the moral concerns of everyday practice. There is also a place for debate about the best approach to the care. This might be patient-specific or policy oriented; either way it is a practical matter, assisted by some theoretical input. When confronted with ethical decisions there is sometimes a temptation to try to convert the problem into a technical one or to characterise it as an organisational matter such that the real nature of the moral question is avoided. If there is a moral question to be confronted, whether it is a *moral choice* or a *dilemma*, it is a judgement that is called for, not a technical fix.

The high-profile complex cases that get into journals and law reports often represent the classic moral dilemma. A *dilemma* is a situation where there is no clear solution, when the alternative courses of action carry disadvantages. A *moral dilemma* is the same except that a moral principle will be compromised whichever course of action is decided upon. A classic, but mercifully rare, example of a moral dilemma is the difficult birth where it is only possible to save either the mother or the baby but not both. Moral arguments can be mounted to support saving the baby and for saving the mother. Each case is sound and can be based on a moral theory. The discussion of a moral dilemma sharpens the debate, makes clear the theories and how they relate to cases. For this reason, ethics is often taught by reference dilemmas. The least worse thing to do is often the best option. Moral choice is much more frequently encountered in daily practice. We should be concerned with the everyday as well as the not so every day moral situations. The moral dilemma is a classic way of approaching a discussion of ethics in health care. It has its uses, it sharpens our views, and allows us to consider cases from various standpoints with the assistance of theories.

In the face of a dilemma, where by definition there is no right way to go, the sides of the argument can be polarised and seem intractable. Moral theories come into their own more obviously here. In the case of the mother, the right to life argument hinges on different principles, a life already in existence, a biography to respect versus the imperative that a newborn helpless infant requires assistance. There is no good answer: this is why it is properly termed a dilemma. Where a solution can be found with no compromise of principle it was not a dilemma in the first place.

It is worth remembering, though, that the moral choices that are made in the practice of nursing have moral concerns and involve principles of rights, justice, respect and so on. The significance of moral choice, because it is more low-key, can be missed. The lowering of standards of care which are found when inquiries are made into hospitals and care homes reveal the obvious lack of attention to the principles which would not sanction the poor care were it planned with concerns for patients' rights and dignity. It is not surprising that some of the worst findings come in hospitals and units where there are organisational difficulties and managerial shortcomings which allow poor practices to persist. These poor practices include patients being left too long waiting for attention; food and drink being delivered and taken away untouched because patients are unable to reach it; and patients in need of personal care being left to their own devices. It would not be true to say that these practices are planned or designed. However, the fact that they are allowed to go unchallenged paves the way for them to become 'acceptable' and so to continue until they are institutionalised and eventually regarded as unavoidable. Everyone involved in such care, including those who find themselves going along with it and perceiving themselves to have neither responsibility for it nor power to do anything about it, has in some way made a moral choice to behave as they do.

There is a difference between a moral judgement and a professional clinical judgement. There will be elements of both in many decisions. The point about ethical debate and the theoretical positions offered by moral philosophy is not to come up with a checklist or rule book. The moral philosopher is concerned to make clear some of the expressions and ideas that we use with less precision than is useful. For example, we speak of something being in the patient's best interests, or being good for them, not always with a clear idea of what this entails, less still with an idea of what the patient would want for themselves. Philosophers spend their time exploring issues; in the case of ethics in practice, exploring moral positions being adopted in relation to various health care matters. They question things that are generally taken as understood or are not questioned at all. The famous statement made by the 4th-century BC Greek philosopher Socrates about the unexamined life not being a life worth living conveys the idea. Alternatively, one might envisage the philosopher as an academic two-year-old, forever asking 'why' and coming to subjects in unexpected ways. The 'why' of the moral philosopher will not be satisfied by the 'because that is how it is' answer of parents and sometimes offered by health care professionals and their institutions. Socrates met his end by a cup of hemlock, having taken his enquiry to the streets of Athens and pursued his quest for understanding of virtue and justice too far for the sensibilities of the day. In 21st-century nursing practice the sharing of information is smiled upon as it generally leads to good outcomes – so a cup of tea is more likely to be the beverage on offer.

The Question that Socrates Asked

Socrates asked 'What sort of person ought one to be?' This question is linked to a second question, 'What ought a good person do?' or 'How ought a good person act?'. These are questions that sustain down the centuries and are as relevant to this book on ethics for nursing and health care practice as they were for Socrates, his pupil Plato and Plato's pupil Aristotle. Campbell et al. say that:

> ethics is best thought of as the critical scrutiny of moral thought and practice. (2005: 2)

They go on to explain:

> For instance, we think it is wrong to kill, as a matter of moral law, but an ethicist would want to know why we think this, whether it is always wrong to kill, and how we justify our conviction of its wrongness in different cases. (2005: 2)

Campbell et al. make clear that Hippocratic thinking remains appropriate today for medical practice, and I would add that it is appropriate too for nursing practice because the focus is on the experience of the patients. As Campbell et al., put it:

> The Hippocratics warned us about becoming captured by theoretical systems, which narrow our thinking about the problems we actually face in real practice, and asked that we substitute reflective intervention and documentation for such theory driven ideologies. (2005: 241)

Aristotle's view was that:

> the qualities that make us human were shown in our thinking, our associations with each other, and our functions as members of the natural order. (Campbell et al., 2005: 3)

This idea has clear resonance with nursing practice. The ways that we relate to patients is the bedrock of care.

Ethical decisions or judgements are not simply theoretical propositions, they must have relevance and meaning in everyday life. The thing about ethics is that it should be a guide to practice. Ethics, Singer tells us, is:

> about how we ought to live what makes an action the right, rather than the wrong thing to do? (1994: 3)

From the discussion so far we can see that ethics and practice belong together. Just as technical competence can be expected of health care professionals, so must there be a consideration of the moral dimension of care. Education for health care professionals includes the clinical aspects of the work, psychosocial concerns and ethics. It is only when all these aspects are brought together that good clinical decisions can be made, decisions which are both clinically and ethically sound. Nursing, as the largest professional group in health care, has to take this proposition to heart.

'Paternalism' is a thing of the past. It is the sociologist's term used to describe that long established way of working in health care where the professionals, usually the doctors, know best and decisions about patient treatment and care are made on behalf of patients. Paternalism has no place in a 21st-century health service. Modern health care is not only characterised by a patient centredness,[6] with the organisation working to meet patients' needs, it is also open and transparent. In other words, patients are given a central position and the National Health Service (NHS) machine should work around this fact.

Is ethics practical or theoretical? Plato's question, as Mayo puts it:

> [W]hat is there about the nature of goodness and rightness which makes it impossible to teach in formal institutions? (1986: 2)

Aristotle, Plato's pupil, thought that virtue (remember, for the ancient Greeks this means an excellence) required to be taught, but that only when a person has gained the knowledge of a virtue practised and then made a habit of it could they become a virtuous person.

Good–Bad and Right–Wrong

Aristotle's question was: 'What is the good life?' A useful distinction is to be made between the ideas of 'good' and 'bad' and between 'right' and 'wrong'. These are not the same thing, even though at first glance good and bad seem to equate with right and wrong. Sometimes, of course, they do equate; for instance, it is wrong to kill and murder is a bad thing. But equivalence is not always the case. Good and bad are graded words, so that nursing practice, for example, can be evaluated along a continuum from *excellent* through *not bad* and *not very good* to *bad*, whereas the notion of right and wrong is about rules and principles being followed or not. Rules are either broken or they are not. The answer to the question 'Is this good or bad?' is not always a clear-cut response, it is not always one or the other. Whilst 'Is this right?' is a different order of question, it is about following rules and the context has a bearing on the answer, but the answer will be 'Yes it is right', or 'No it is wrong'. It is one or the other, rather like a test for pregnancy: it is positive or negative – it is not possible to be a little bit pregnant.

Mayo makes the helpful point that right–wrong, good–bad (or good–evil)

> are not interchangeable. 'Right' and 'wrong' apply primarily to actions. 'Good' and 'bad' or 'evil' apply much more widely, to states of affairs, to people, to characters, to motives. (1986: 40)

---

[6]The idea of putting the patient in the centre was the main organising theme of the Labour government's modernised NHS started in 1997 (DH, 2000).

To give an example we could say that to feed someone is generally speaking a good thing to do. If, however, that person is about to undergo a general anaesthetic, it would be the wrong thing to do. That is to say it would not be the 'right' thing to do. So in such a case 'right' and 'good' are not the same thing. Likewise thumping someone on the chest is a bad thing to do. However, if that person's heart has just stopped, it would be the right thing to do. This does not make generalised thumping of people on the chest a good thing, it is still generally a bad thing. However, in certain circumstances it is the right, and not the wrong, thing to do.

Mayo (1986: 40) describes two kinds of criteria against which to judge something, a criterion being something we use to judge things by. There are two different kinds of criteria against which we judge a thing. First, there is the criterion called a *standard* which Mayo says:

enables us to make judgements in a continuous range or scale, using terms such as 'good', or 'poor', 'mediocre', 'excellent' and so on. (1986: 84)

Standards of care are required of a qualified nurse, for example. Second, there is the criterion of judgement which is a *principle* or *rule*:

[T]he judgement is not of the 'more or less' kind, but of the 'yes or no' kind such as a verdict. (Mayo, 1986: 84)

When rules or principles are the criteria of judgement then the judgement is not a graded one; in other words, the answer is not a very good, average, poor and so on kind of answer, it is a 'yes' or 'no' answer, 'yes' or 'no' because rules or principles either prescribe or proscribe, they say this is what should be done and that should not be done (proscribe). So when the criteria used for judging nursing care are the principles of beneficence (to do good) and non-maleficence (to do no harm), the judgement is not about nearly doing good or not doing much harm: the judgement is about whether the principle or rule has been obeyed or not obeyed. This is all very relevant to care and standards of care. In ethics for nursing practice we are interested in the morality of actions and also the character of the nurse. We return to this in later chapters. For the moment it is helpful to get these distinctions straight.

Whether something is right or wrong is conditional on the context. For example, it is not wrong to have a drink on some occasions, but the same action would be wrong in others. Driving, being on duty or being engaged in some other activity in which drinking is not a wise thing to do, are instances of occasions where drinking would be wrong. With right and wrong we are talking about following rules and laws or guidelines. These examples are fairly straightforward as there are clear contraindications in these situations. There are other areas of life where it is not so easy to say what is right or wrong. A generalised way of looking at this is to consider the distinction between what 'is' (fact) and what 'ought' (value) to be. To talk about what 'ought' to be is to employ a value judgement. The distinctions are between 'is' the situation that exists, which is a matter of 'fact', and 'ought', which is the expression of a desirable state of affairs, a value. For example, to say that there are no empty beds in the hospital this evening is a statement of fact. To state that the Health Trust ought to ensure that there are always beds available for emergency admissions is to express an aspiration based on a value of justice. Or to take a rather more individual-level example of the difference between 'is' and 'ought', patients are sometimes treated badly – fact; health care professionals should always treat people with respect – value. This 'ought' statement is aspirational and might be based on the principle of respect for autonomy, or on the basis of the notion of rights.

The link between the two, between *is* and *ought*, is what Mayo calls 'a trouble-some contrast':

> [G]enerally speaking, the facts are not what they should be, and what ought to be is not in fact the case; what ought not to be all too often is. (1986: 3)

A rather gloomy view, but it makes the point. This gap between the 'is' and the 'ought' is a puzzle. Philosophers since the ancient Greek times have debated the question of how life should be lived, what one 'ought' to do to live the good life. Philosophical ideas and religious beliefs are intertwined and so we are left with a rich heritage of philosophical theory and religious teachings available to us when we study and seek to justify the rights and wrongs of human behaviour. It is Aristotle's work[7] on ethics to which we still look in the context of today's ethics for health care practice.

Introduction to the Rest of the Book

This makes a good point at which to introduce the content of the chapters.

Chapter 2 introduces the main principles that lie at the root of ethical debates in health care. The four-principles approach shows how most moral debates come down to the four principles of beneficence, non-maleficence, respect for persons (autonomy) and justice.

In *Chapter 3* the sociological perspective is introduced to show how ethical debate in nursing and health care, whilst led by moral philosophy, does not take place in a moral vacuum but rather in the rather chaotic world of clinical reality. Individual conscience theory is explored in *Chapter 4*; this is to demonstrate that we need something less subjective than individual conscience theory for professional ethics.

---

[7]Aristotle's *Nicomachean Ethics*, so called as it was produced by Aristotle's son, Nicomachus, is one of the most influential works in moral philosophy. The translation used in this book is Thomson (1976).

Adam Smith's idea of the 'impartial spectator' is introduced as a more objective approach to right and wrong. In *Chapter 5* Kantian or duty-based theory rests on the idea that acting according to one's duty and obligations will bring about the best for society. *Chapter 6* is concerned with the legal context of nursing practice and the relationship between law and ethics. *Chapter 7* discusses utilitarianism – greatest good theory. This is a consequentialist theory, propounded by Jeremy Bentham and John Stuart Mill.

Chapter 8 looks at rights-based ethics, which fits well with the 21st-century approach to health care. *Chapter 9* is about virtue ethics and its links to professional regulation. In *Chapter 10* the main themes of the book are drawn together, with a focus on trust.

- Morals are values and associated rules and practices by which people live; ethics – also called moral philosophy – is concerned with the study of morality.
- With right and wrong we are talking about following rules and laws or guidelines, whereas good and bad are graded words.
- Aristotle's idea of *habituation* means doing something repeatedly so that it becomes second nature – a habit. Aristotle held that 'moral virtues, like crafts, are acquired by practice and habituation'.
- Many of our ideas about ethics come from the Greeks and have a contemporary ring to them.

2

Principles at the Root of Ethical Debate

It may seem a strange principle to enunciate as the very first requirement in a Hospital that it should do the sick no harm.

Florence Nightingale, 1863

The aim of this chapter is to introduce four main principles that can be said to lie at the root of ethical debates in health care. Beauchamp and Childress, leading figures in bioethics,[1] are the authors most associated with what have become known within medical ethics as 'the four principles'. These are: beneficence, non-maleficence, respect for autonomy and justice.

Beneficence means to do good, and along with it goes the principle of *non-maleficence*, to do no harm. This second principle has a long history going all the way back to Hippocrates.[2] *Respect for autonomy* is also expressed as 'respect for persons': this is the basic principle which underpins individual liberty and the right that people have to conduct their lives as they see fit, with due respect for the rights of others. *Justice* is essentially the idea that people should be treated fairly. Fairness is a complex idea: it does not simply mean treating everyone alike. However, justice is a strong principle which, despite its complexity, in practice carries a clear message.

The four principles serve as a framework to shape, or at least bring some order to, ethical debate and help to steer a course through the complex terrain of moral philosophy.

---

[1]Beauchamp and Childress (2001); this is an American text and 'biomedical ethics' is used in the US where we would more commonly say 'medical ethics'.

[2]It is part of the Hippocratic Oath, which is still taken at graduation ceremonies in medical schools across the world.

'Principlism' is the rather unattractive term sometimes used to describe this approach, which advocates basing ethical debate on four fundamental principles. These four principles occur in the more specific ethical theories and their attraction is that they provide a basis for practical ethical debate and offer a means of engaging in discussion of individual cases in need of practical solutions, without becoming overly caught up in ethical theory.

In order to state the moral argument in a case, the discussion necessarily becomes theoretical. This can be off-putting for the newcomer to ethics as it can convey the idea that all of the available moral theories have to be digested before we can embark upon ethical debate, whereas the four principles can convey a general feel for ethical debate – a soundly based feel as these principles lie at the root of ethical theories.

The four principles approach is also useful because it gives an unrestricted view of the different kinds of justification for moral decisions and actions. This approach recognises that ethics is not about adopting this or that theory and disregarding others in the process of moral reasoning. According to Beauchamp and Childress:

> 'the top' (principles and theories) and 'the bottom' (cases, individual judgements) are not solely sufficient for biomedical ethics. Neither general principles nor paradigm cases have sufficient power to generate conclusions ... Principles need to be made specific for cases, and case analysis needs illumination from general principles. (2001: 397)

Gillon says in praise of the four-principles approach to practical ethics that it:

> offers a transcultural, transnational, trans-religious, trans-philosophical framework for ethical analysis; that it offers elements of a common language for such ethical analysis ... Because it is not itself a theory, but instead draws on elements common to most if not all moral theories, it can function peaceably as a tool of practical ethics that may be shared by those whose theories are totally incompatible and antithetical. (1994: 332)

Casuistry – Principles and Individual Cases

It is worth taking a brief look at casuistry. 'Casuistry' is the term that refers to a way of thinking and reasoning that involves trying to apply moral rules to particular cases. Beauchamp and Childress define casuistry in these terms:

> Casuistry refers to the use of case comparison and analogy to reach moral conclusions. (2001: 392)

Casuistry is not always included in discussions of ethics in nursing and medicine. However, I think that it is of interest because it raises some of the concerns that sociological analysis of ethical cases highlight, in terms of context and an understanding of the ways that people behave in the situations that give rise to moral questions in practice.

Toulmin (1981), who has written of 'the tyranny of principles', says that casuists do not like rules and general theories because they leave aside context and specifics of the case.

Gillon makes this useful comment on casuistry:

> Casuistry is then the application of general ethical principles to particular cases. Under a different guise this is also the basis of the case law approach to English law. The four principles as a set of general *prima facie* moral principles are entirely compatible with casuistry which seeks to apply them to particular cases. (1994: 327)

Like Aristotle, the casuist would argue that the rights and wrongs of a case should be determined bearing the facts of the individual circumstances and specific situation in mind. There have been periods in which casuistry fell into disrepute, such as during the Reformation when it was linked to compromises with church teachings, and again in modern times when 'casuistry' had come to mean false or even dodgy reasoning. However, recently, through the work of its main protagonists Jonsen and Toulmin (1988), interest in casuistry has been revived. Beauchamp and Childress (2001: 393) accuse Jonsen and Toulmin of having done some damage to the four principles approach during their efforts to rehabilitate casuistry. Beauchamp and Childress maintain that Jonsen and Toulmin 'have, in the process criticised our framework of principles'.

So all is not sweetness and light even in the garden of moral philosophy!

The usefulness of the four principles approach can be seen in this example:

> A classic dilemma was the subject of the play *Whose Life is it Anyway?*,[3] staged in London in the 1980s, that told a very poignant tale of a young man who wanted his life to end and the hospital staff who saw every reason not to go along with his wishes. The leading character in the play is a sculptor who is rendered quadriplegic in a road accident. He has retained all his mental faculties and decides that he wants to be allowed to die.
>
> In one memorable scene one of the doctors refuses to accept that 'a man of Harrison's intelligence would choose suicide'. The second doctor points out that this is exactly what he has done. To which the first doctor replies, 'Therefore he is unbalanced'. The theme of the play is conflict between the right to autonomy, the right to control one's own life and the professional's duty to preserve life where possible. The power of the drama lies in the fact that you are gradually persuaded by the sculptor and are on his side; and the doctors and nurses emerge as the 'bad guys'. There is dramatic licence and few would find themselves caught up in such a case, but the issues are real enough. The point is that such a dramatic and polarised dilemma allows the debate to cover the principles involved, even though the solution is going to lie in compromise.

---

[3] A novel by David Benedictus (1982) based on a play by Brian Clark.

Respect for persons is clearly in play here.

This book is essentially about practice but the political context cannot be avoided. Take the example of the Trust manager who was a whistle-blower:[4]

> A recent case is an NHS Trust manager who chose to follow the ethical code and speak out about poor standards and to ignore the so-called gagging clause that he had signed as part of a severance package ending his contract with the NHS Trust. These clauses, of doubtful legality, are agreements that employees are required to sign by which they agree not to speak about the agreement or their reasons for leaving. In this case the Trust manager went to the press to talk about the effects on patient care of following government targets rather than clinical need.
>
> The individual who gets caught up in these whistle-blowing scenarios sets out to do their duty – in this case to draw attention to poor standards of hospital care. The code of conduct requires them to do this, and at risk is their self-interest and their salary, which is theirs by right.

All of the four principles are involved here. The whistle-blower considered the patients' interests: beneficence and non-maleficence. As for the poor care standards, the underlying principles are respect for persons and justice. In this example the choice that the Trust faced was to focus on clinical priorities as expressed by the clinicians or to meet government targets. The two may not always match; the government seeks to reduce waiting lists for non-urgent surgery to meet their election manifesto pledges. There is pressure on beds for urgent cases, typically in the winter months. The clinical imperative is to focus on these short-term needs and as a consequence the waiting lists would remain, in the government's view, unacceptably long. The Trust opted to follow government policy and had therefore to ensure that the clinicians' views were overridden.

It is worth noting that the legalistic approach to whistle-blowing is not the way to serve the best interests of patients. The problems need to be aired in an open and transparent system rather than through legal measures and the bearers of bad news being paid off and silenced.

Whatever the ethical theory being drawn upon, Beauchamp and Childress (2001: 12) say that these principles can be found as fundamental parts of the arguments. The four ethical principles, they argue, can be employed in ethical debate, whatever the substantive issue in question. On this analysis, whilst the ethical issues and clinical cases may differ in detail, they maintain that the underlying ethical principles and positions are the same and can, for the most part, be traced back to the four principles.

---

[4]'Whistle-blowing' is the term used for health care professionals who speak out usually about poor care standards; when this happens it is an embarrassment for managers and can be associated with so-called 'gagging clauses' being introduced into NHS Foundation Trust Hospital contracts.

- The four principles serve as a framework to shape ethical debate.
- The principles work across ethical theories and enable practical reasoning and ethical debate.
- The importance of transparency.
- Whistle-blowing should be a thing of the past.

3

Nursing and Health Care Ethics – the Sociological Perspective

Jaques: I do not like her name.

Orlando: There was no thought of pleasing you when she was christened.

Shakespeare, c.1600, *As You Like It*, III, ii

A view of nursing – overheard in a coffee shop in Edinburgh[1]

Two women, sitting a couple of tables away from me, were discussing visiting a friend in hospital. The friend had complained that the place was noisy. They went on to speak about their own experiences of noise in wards at night. Their discussion was lively and with much laughter. One said that she had been kept awake by nurses chatting, laughing and generally making noise at the nurses' station all through the night. Her friend laughed and said that at the hospital that she has experience of they were too short-staffed for that kind of thing to go on. The first woman continued with her tale of the noisy ward, repeating with increasing laughter and volume, 'and this was four in the morning!'. She had been woken by the nurse who said sorry to disturb her but she had forgotten to ask her what she wanted for her breakfast. She went on to say that the nurse had then asked about lunch. The woman said that she had told the nurse

---

[1] I would like to say that I made this up as an illustration, but I am afraid I cannot!

that she did not intend still being there at lunchtime as she was an overnight stay case, but the nurse with the incomplete breakfast order had persisted. Both women were now laughing and repeating in unison 'and this was four in the morning!'. More laughter and then the teller of the story continued, yes, and the nurse had reeled off hot dishes from the menu, 'remember, this is four in the morning!' she said, laughing now, though probably not then. By now a good number of people in the coffee shop were laughing. I concentrated on my newspaper.

Nurses do not come out of this story particularly well. There is a fairly good-humoured acceptance of their behaviour, and it makes a good story. From a professional point of view, it is not such a good story and not the image that nurses would really want to have. In the situation described, surely the better course of action would have been for the nurse to fill in the menu order sheet: that is, to tell a written white lie and let the patient sleep. A more urgent need for information would be worth waking a patient for. It is a matter of balance between doing good and doing harm.

This conversation can run as a cautionary tale through the chapters of this book. We could refer back to it like a running joke, were it not so damning. Nonetheless, it makes a good point about the social context in which nursing takes place. It also illustrates the power of audit and form filling, and what has been called 'mindless bureaucracy'. Presumably the nurse thought that she was going to make it difficult for the patient to get breakfast and lunch without the requisite paperwork. Maybe her belief in patient autonomy and the right to choose her own food trumped the right to a good night's sleep.

Nursing takes place in the public gaze. There is the particular clinical work setting in which a nurse is practising where those cared for and their friends and relatives can have a view on what goes on. Also there is the wider backdrop against which nursing takes place – this is in the climate of public opinion. Nurses, generally speaking, enjoy a good public image; however, in the wake of difficulties and outright scandals that occur from time to time attracting full media coverage, the professional image and reputation suffers.

The practice of nursing is a complex business, where there are many competing demands. Every organisation has its systems and protocols, designed to ensure the smooth running of the organisation. The central focus is on the patient, with the professionals, management and general bureaucracy working to that end. This is very much part of the process of modernising the NHS (DH, 2000). The tale of the menu in the night, aside from being an example of an unintended consequence of having systems which are not sufficiently flexible, tells us something of how far a reach these well intended systems have and illustrates the point that individual judgement still has its place.

In cases where the problems are a good deal more serious, the response has to be more than a 'that's life' kind of shrug. Various commissions and reports followed the publication in February 2011 of *Care and Compassion?*, the report by the

Parliamentary and Health Service Ombudsman, which exposed shocking failures in the care of older people.[2]

Another example of a more serious unintended consequence was the public reaction to the use of the Liverpool Care Pathway (LCP).[3]

> The Marie Curie Foundation and Liverpool University designed a care pathway (LCP) with the intention of improving end-of-life care and to avoid unnecessary intervention when a patient is dying. Its production was in response to complaints about too much aggressive intervention in the end stages of life. It became the subject of media attention and a number of relatives complaining that hospitals were using the LCP in order to hasten deaths and so empty (so-called) blocked beds. Worse still, the press linked these complaints to the Department of Health financial incentives for Health Trusts improving end-of-life care. The press version was, crudely put, that the government was paying Trusts to hasten the end of patients' lives by use of the LCP. It was portrayed as a care plan which involved no nutrition and no fluid and so was regarded as an unacceptable practice. The facts of the matter are that the LCP is implemented in a carefully monitored way and whilst cessation of nutrition and hydration is part of the plan, in order to allow the patient to be more comfortable, any sign that nutrition and fluids were indicated, then they would be given. The perception of the relatives of some patients was that the pathway was set and followed come what may, whilst others had nothing but praise for the care of their relative at the end of life and were pleased that the LCP had been followed.

Despite the fact that one of the key principles of the LCP is that, 'it neither hastens nor postpones death', such was the public controversy and confused debate around the LCP that the government Minister for Care and Support commissioned an independent review, chaired by the crossbench peer, Baroness Neuberger. The report[4] was published in July 2013 and among many recommendations was an important one that, 'the name "Liverpool Care Pathway" should be abandoned'. The rationale being that, 'An "end of life care plan" should be sufficient for both professionals and lay people'. (p53)

The recommendations in the Neuberger report are essentially in line with the LCP where the original aim was, 'to improve care of the dying in the last days and hours of life.'

---

[2]In February 2012 the Commission on Dignity in Care for Older People published its draft report, *Delivering Dignity*, for consultation.

[3]Liverpool Care Pathway for the Dying Patient was developed by the Marie Curie Palliative Care Institute and Liverpool University as a means of achieving well co-ordinated care at the end of life (www.mcpcil.org.uk).

[4]Independent Review of the Liverpool Care Pathway (2013) *More Care, Less Pathway – A Review of the Liverpool Care Pathway*. Available at www.gov.uk/dh (accessed 15 July 2013).

The term 'pathway' was probably never helpful, but the main problems with the LCP were the misunderstandings and media coverage which represented it as an authoritarian approach to care which left no room for professional judgement and patient involvement: the mainstays of clinical practice. The Neuberger report provides a useful counterpoint to the unintended consequences of the LCP and demonstrates the on-going nature of ethical debate.

Nurses and other health care professionals in their attempts to follow the guidance of health care ethics have to make the best of the clinical situation in which they find themselves. Ethical theories and the moral arguments which can be mounted as frameworks of principles serve to enable the ethical discussion. Importantly, the clinical situation, the context, has to be taken into account. So when nurses are making decisions in conjunction, whenever this is possible, with the patient, they have in mind the patient's best interests. Ethical debates and legal considerations provide a sound backdrop to those decisions and play a useful role in arriving at the judgements made. Remembering Aristotle's view that ethics is a practical matter, we have to recognise that unless ethics relates to practical situations, the debates are of no real use. The clinical world is one of messy compromise and negotiation and is always unpredictable and uncertain. Clinical decisions – be they the larger ones which approach dilemma proportions or the lesser but important matters of day-to-day moral choice – have to be worked out in the context of the care setting.

This chapter is concerned with the wider context within which nursing takes place and how this affects practice. The wider context also has implications for ethics for nursing practice. Sociological analysis gives us some understanding of the way that health care works in practice. Philosophical theories and principles have their place and, as we have seen in Chapter 2, they provide a basis upon which to make decisions about the right or best thing to do when we are confronted in practice with difficult choices. An understanding of organisations, the relationship between professionals and patients and wider social considerations helps us to set ethical decision making into a more practical perspective. For instance, a focus on autonomy and the primacy of patients' rights to do as they wish leaves out of the equation the demands of others in the system. Ethical debate in nursing is, of course, led by moral philosophy and the principles that underpin good practice. However, the clinical world is a rather uncertain place and clinical realities are somewhat less ordered than a philosophical approach allows. The important point here is that ethical debate, driven as it is by moral philosophical principles, does not take place in a moral vacuum. It takes place in the rather messy clinical reality that is health care.

Sociology and Ethics – Explanation of the Context of Practice

Sociology is concerned, among other things, with understanding how society and groups within society work. It includes study of social institutions such as the family, marriage and partnership, organisations and bureaucracies and so on. Nearer to our interests here, medical sociology (or more properly, sociology of health and ill-ness) concerns itself with health and illness, the health care professions, the work-ings of organisations and work places and the health service. This is not a sociology text and so we are not overly concerned with its methods; rather it is a consideration of its insights and their utility in terms of understanding nursing practice that is of interest. It is, however, worth noting in passing that the methods of sociology differ from those of philosophy mainly in the fact that sociology makes use of data. Data are the product of observation and other means of acquiring information – interviews, diary keeping, records, archives and statistics.

In the case of nursing, sociological data can range from statistical information to qualitative data. For instance, the numbers of patients nursed by how many nurses, along with patient dependency data, are used in workforce studies. Qualitative data afford insights into the nature of practice and the communication between pro-fessionals and patients. There is a distinction to be made between *empirical* work, which draws upon data, and *theoretical* work, which starts from what we know and sets out a 'theory' or proposed explanation. The difference between theoretical and empirical work lies in the dependency on data in empirical research, whereas theo-retical work is more abstract and conceptual.

This book is concerned with the ethical issues which arise in the everyday practice of nursing. Almost every aspect of nursing has a moral dimension. In this chapter we seek to demonstrate the wider social context in which these moral concerns are played out.

Edinburgh café bar conversation

This was a chance overhearing of a conversation in a public place. It included, surprisingly, questions for ethics for nursing practice and more widely for ethics in health care. I became aware of this conversation at the next table when I heard someone say 'do not resuscitate'. I paused, as ironically I was at the time revising a draft section of this book, so the ethics reference caught my ear. As I gave the conversation my full attention I heard, 'I want to be comfortable when I'm dying – I don't want to die in a rush'. This, it struck me, was a very down-to-earth everyday expression of a moral choice. It held nothing of the attendant chill of the increasingly common media debates (BBC Radio 4, *Newsnight*) about the right to determine when death will come about. Another phrase that wafted over to my table was, 'If by any chance you happened to die of morphine, that was alright'.

This café bar rendering of the principle of double effect[5] was as attention-grabbing as the memorable line about not dying in a rush. It reminds us that ethical debate about nursing and health care, whilst informed by moral philosophy, does not take

---

[5]The double effect of morphine, relief of pain and shortening of life. The aim of relieving pain should not be thwarted because of the attendant shortening of life. The morality lies in the intention, not the consequence.

place in a moral vacuum. Rather it takes place in a social context, where open debate of health and the practice of its professions are open to public scrutiny, opinion and misunderstandings. This conversation, whilst it sounded as casual as a discussion about the weather, touched on two very fundamental concerns of those interested in ethics for practice. It also is an example of moral choice and very possibly dilemma. The expression of the wish not to 'die in a rush', mentioned alongside a very oblique reference to the principle of the double effect in relation to morphine, put this conversation firmly in the territory of health care ethics.

Decisions Concerning Resources

Sociology as a discipline is concerned with explaining the social world and the ways in which society organises its activity through social institutions, such as the family, marriage, education. In this book we are interested in the organisation of health care and nursing practice within that health care system. The sociological perspective offers an analysis of the context in which nursing takes place and concerns itself with the study of nursing practices and understanding how care is produced.

Ethical debate has to recognise the context: for example, the way that nurses allocate their time to patients might appear to be a matter of logistics, but there is an element of choice involved. When staffing levels are low and getting through the work is difficult, the freedom to choose how to allocate time does not reside in the clinical area. Nurses working in such conditions are more or less left having to manage as best they can. However, the decisions made further up the system, whether they are in hospital management or government departments, as to which resources will be made available, are the result of a choice of one sort or another.

The distinction we have seen between a moral dilemma and a moral choice is a useful one to assist in this discussion. The choices that we make have consequences, but they are often not of dilemma proportions: that is to say, where principles are compromised, whichever decision is taken they are nonetheless important. When it comes to resources, the moral dimension comes in the results of choices made. These consequences sometimes only become apparent in the clinical settings, where the impact is inescapable. A shortage of beds can lead to patients spending time in areas of the hospital which are not equipped to handle their needs. This is an organisational problem, to an extent, and the solution lies in the structures, policies and management. These are also ethical questions to raise in clinical, managerial and political terms.

Clinical Governance

All of this does not detract from the practical ethical matter of what to do on the ward, or indeed in the corridor, at the time. Nurses are expected to care for their patients in appropriate, competent and ethically sound ways. So how should these situations, where conditions are not ideal, play out in the clinical reality of the ward?

Recognising the organisational extent of responsibility for the care patients receive does not mean that individual nurses can ignore the moral choices about where to place their effort and time with patients when there is some scope for discretion. The idea of clinical governance[6] covers this joint responsibility for the quality of care.

Sociological analysis can demonstrate how systems work and how people fare in them. In the case of the NHS the focus of sociological analysis has been on the professions, on patients and often on interaction between the two groups (e.g. Allen, 2001; Atkinson, 1995; Friedson, 1970; Melia, 1987). Also there is a considerable body of work on the nature of professions in health care and studies of the place of professions in organisations. Traditionally, professions could be described as a sub-set of occupations which have certain privileges in work organisation by virtue of the specialist knowledge that they possess and offer to the organisation. The rise of managerialism and a focus on consumer opinion – in the health service, patients are sometimes characterised as consumers – has caused some to question the position that professions now hold in the hierarchy of occupations and within the organisation of work. Health service managers determining the priorities and setting financial targets for clinical work is an example of this shift in the balance of power. An example is priority being given to reducing the length of waiting lists for cold surgery at the expense of activity driven by clinical decisions and priorities of the doctors and nurses.

Freidson (2001) has a particularly useful analysis of professions and the sociology of applied knowledge (i.e. the study of specialist knowledge of the professionals in health care as opposed to the contribution of the non-clinical managers). He makes the case for professionalism: that is, the ideology which describes the methods employed by the professions whereby the status of the professional is justified on the basis of their specialised knowledge and control over their professional activity.

The third logic of Freidson's work is the professional model of work organisation. For the professions, work is the practical application of knowledge, our interests here being in nursing and medicine. There are various approaches to work and associated sources of control. Freidson describes three types of work organisation: free market consumerism, bureaucratic managerialism and professionalism. The special status of *professionalism* as an ideology is made clear if we contrast it to the alternatives or opposing ideologies that Freidson describes, namely, managerialism and consumerism. *Consumerism* is the idea that it is the market that controls the health care system, based on the notion that the customers know what they want. *Managerialism* operates through a bureaucratic organisation, where roles and responsibilities are defined in a system designed to run without regard to the individuals occupying the roles. Competent and appropriately qualified individuals must occupy the roles, but beyond that the system runs without regard for the details of the individuals in the role. Bureaucracies run according to roles and responsibilities, rules and lines of authority. They are designed specifically to run without paying heed to the individuals: the focus is on role and function.

Freidson accepts that few occupations can be truly fully in control of their work, particularly when they operate within organisations. The workings of the health care

---

[6]Clinical governance is the corporate responsibility for quality of care – the idea being that everyone involved in the organisation has a part to play in ensuring quality.

marketplace, the loosening up of medical dominance and an increasing emphasis on patient-centred care all feature in this change in the ideology which is in place in the health service. In short, it is a shift away from professionalism towards managerialism.

Unintended Consequences

A not infrequent finding of the sociological studies of health care is that original intentions of the policy and organisational protocols do not produce the intended outcomes. The unintended consequences of the best laid plans are to an extent inevitable. They are, however, worth considering, and the practical ethics approach can help. The four main principles described by Beauchamp and Childress (2001), as we saw in Chapter 2, are a useful start here as they cover most eventualities. Alongside the practicalities of the situation, they provide a basis from which to consider consequences for patients.

The contributions of moral philosophical insights and sociological analysis allow an examination of clinical practice in the context of professional cultures and every-day work situations. Moral philosophers tend to move back and forth between individual illustrative cases and their theoretical propositions and ethical principles, whereas sociologists attempt to understand the situation as it is and will therefore tend to have some empirical basis to their studies. It is really a bit of a caricature to say that philosophers are interested in real cases, 'facts', only in so far as they illustrate their arguments, just as it is too simplistic to say that sociologists dismiss ethical debate as someone else's business rather than taking it on as a necessary part of their enterprise. There is, however, a grain of truth in these caricatures. The sociological approach to the study of health care often has a moral dimension to the work and differs from philosophy in the emphasis that it places on data. We should not hesitate to combine the two, moral philosophy and sociology, if a more useful analysis results.

For example, take a busy medical ward in which it is being made difficult to work and unpleasant to experience as a patient because of the very noisy and disruptive behaviour of a few 'demanding' patients. Nurses might attempt to respond to the demands until time, patience and capacity to continue in that way run out and they resort to ignoring these patients. Having satisfied themselves that there is no obvious clinical problem and certainly no danger, they avoid the patients until the rest of ward's needs have been met. In taking this not altogether unreasonable line the nurses create a further problem for themselves and their patients. The nurses are feeling pressured first by the noise and second by the strain of ignoring it. Other patients cannot see why order is not restored, and whilst appreciating that they are being cared for, the situation is likely to raise questions in their minds about the professionalism and possibly the

(Continued)

(Continued)

competence of the nursing staff. By visiting time some order may be restored, but the demanding patients continue to disrupt. Now the situation is viewed by visitors who may also draw conclusions about the standards of care and attitude of the nursing staff and maybe blame the hospital, the ward or the individual nurses.

Explanations for such a situation can be various, and I am not suggesting that a sociological study be instigated. However, sociological literature and workforce studies in hospitals can tell us something about the effects that staffing levels and skill mix can have on the smooth running of patient care. Staffing levels are not the only consideration; some patients require a different kind of care requiring different skills. If, as is increasingly the case, there is a shortage of beds in the long-term care sector, or there is a delay in planned discharges because community services are stretched at certain times of the year, there can be beds 'blocked' (an unfortunate term, with attendant ethical issues of its own) by patients whose needs are not easily met in acute settings. It is also possible that the admission of patients to acute beds, where their needs are going to put a strain on that setting, causes similar problems. The system, in other words, is creating problems for those trying to work within it.

These kinds of tensions are never an excuse for bad practice or care which falls short of the ethical principles upon which it is based. However, simply to state that there is no excuse for bad practice does not solve the problem because we are dealing with human beings and so the care they produce and receive is affected by these organisational factors. Human beings do respond, both well and badly, to different circumstances. The kinds of circumstances described here can be temporary; they may be dealt with and everyone moves on. They may, however, escalate and produce more critical outcomes. Or, and this seems the most likely, they persist in a low-key fashion which is generally 'coped with', but as a consequence expectations, standards and behaviours change over time, eventually producing a situation which is not satisfactory but is somehow tolerated. Tolerated, that is, until either a crisis occurs or complaints eventually come about through whistle-blowers or friends of the patient making an official complaint. Either way the media and press are also often involved.

The reactions of the relatives of the patients who died whilst in the care of the Mid Staffordshire NHS Foundation Trust can serve as a backdrop to the discussion. Suffice it to say here that the social context of care described by the Inquiry (Francis, 2013), included concerns about organisation, staffing levels and public perspective. All of this provides a background against which to have the debate about ethics for nursing practice. The end point of such situations is clearly and shockingly described in the *Independent Inquiry into Care Provided by Mid Staffordshire NHS Foundation Trust* (Francis, 2013). Sadly, this is not the only such report, although it must be remembered that these occurrences are relatively rare. Rarity is not a precise term and one such case is one too many, so any insights that we can gain from them have to be taken seriously. We must always be alert to the possibility that similar, but undiscovered, instances exist. Indeed, the Keough Review[7] (2013) following on from the Mid Staffordshire Inquiry found other trusts with 'significant scope for improvement with some urgent needs to be addressed to raise the standards of care'. Keogh characterises the problem, saying 'these organisations have been trapped in mediocrity'. The review is written in a refreshingly realistic and optimistic way, expressing the recommendations in terms of 'achievable ambitions'.

Lessons Learned

The delivery and organisation of nursing care is a complex business and when things go wrong the answers are not simple. However, it often appears to outsiders to be the case that the answers are simple, and sometimes they may have a point. Why isn't basic care carried out? How was that person left to fall? Why wasn't that person helped to eat their lunch? Why are patients left on trolleys for so long? It all seems so easy. So when there are problems, the reactions that follow range from quick knee-jerk answers of politicians and the glib news items. Random demands and edicts from government departments about smiling and caring: reactions sometimes lead all the way to Public Inquiries and Commissions. At the time all of these responses seem, at least to some, to be the answer. Yet they also seem to miss the point.

This is too gloomy a view in some ways, but consider the number of times we hear 'Lessons must be learnt' following a damning inquiry, and it might lead us to ask more questions. If the answers were easy, the problems would not be so persistent. Answers are not going to be found listed in a book such as this. However, a good start can be made by recognising that the response has to be a steady, consistent concern with these matters. And that whilst money is by no means always the answer, a properly financed and staffed health service working in conjunction with a comprehensive social care system would provide the foundation for safe and ethical health and social care.

The social context of the official inquiries and public criticism of nursing along with the nature of the media coverage have an effect on the responses from both the profession and the government. Senior members of the profession do not always help matters when their response is rather supine in the face of the criticism. Taking a transparent leadership and clinical managerial stand to make clear the extent of the problem without complacency and to make explicit what is to happen next is the approach needed. An over-readiness on the part of government to take criticism at face value and to extrapolate from the problem area right across the service is

---

[7]Professor Bruce Keogh (July 2013) *Review into the Quality of Care and Treatment Provided by 14 Hospital Trusts in England: Overview Report.* NHS. Available at www.nhs.uk/ NHSEngland/bruce-keogh-review

unhelpful, not least because it creates a climate of mistrust in the health service and demonises large numbers of health care professionals who are continuing to do a good job. A longer-term view would tell us that a demoralised workforce is not going to be up to the job and there will be consequential effects on recruitment and retention of staff.

So what to do in situations like the one at Mid Staffordshire? Jumping to conclusions, calling for prosecutions and fast fixes are not the solution. Any immediate action which would help is, of course, imperative. But the danger of too quick a generalised response is that only the symptoms are treated and the causes left to work another day. The one approach need not preclude the other, and of course any action to stop the harm must be an immediate priority. Longer-term answers lie in gaining an understanding of why this kind of thing is happening and so compromising care. There is often a call for a culture change with perhaps little regard for the complexity and long-term nature of such change. Freidson rejects the term 'culture change' as a 'formless catch-all term which can refer to almost anything'. He says that:

> ideology can be used more precisely to designate elements of culture which are thought to provide authoritative explanation and justification for a particular set of institutions like professionalism. (2001: 106n1)

Ethical debate conducted away from the cut and thrust of daily practice must be incorporated as an essential part of planning and organising nursing practice. Debates about why we do things, and about how we are going to make the system work and continue to work, are the stuff of ethics for nursing practice. Any occurrence in practice has to be understood in the context in which it happened.

> For instance, one of the complaints often made in cases of sub-standard care is that call bells go unanswered. If a number of bells go at once, it is going to be the case that there will be delays. But if there are deeper organisational reasons for calls going unanswered routinely, and moreover that it is not perceived to be a bad thing, then there is a case to answer.

The longer-term solutions lie in education, appropriately skilled staff and standards.

The Perceived Image of the Nursing Profession

There is a public image of nursing, and most people think that they know what nursing is about. There is a climate in which everyone feels free to comment on nursing and its practice. We see examples of this when the government has no hesitation in suggesting ideas about how nursing should work. It is hard to imagine other professions being dispensed such unsolicited advice. This idea that everyone supposes that they understand what nursing is about includes government Ministers of the Crown. There have been other initiatives, including the advice that nurses should smile more often! It does not help to confuse familiarity with compassion. This would indeed be something to smile about if it were not indicative of the difficult position that it puts nursing in. The issues are more deep-seated and lie in the organisational context within which nursing takes place. If we are going to have a service which takes respect for patients as a given, nurses, smiling or not, need sufficient time to undertake the work and a work organisation which allows freedom to develop professional relationships with patients.

The image of nursing as a profession in disarray is fed by the publication of stories such as the one that made the national press when a patient made a 999 call because he could not get an answer to his bell call for water. Of course, the press should report; however, sometimes journalists' rather lazy analysis and eye-catching headlines can end up appearing to be ready criticism of nursing as a whole. However, it is sometimes forgotten that this makes the situation difficult for all nurses who have to continue to provide the service until truths are discovered and remedial action taken. The Allitt[8] case stands as a symbol of all that can go wrong with nursing, in much the same way that the case of the serial killer Harold Shipman was a landmark in the professional regulation of medicine. These are plainly the dramatic and the rare cases; much more common are the daily moral issues which arise and whilst not having the shock effect that the criminal cases have, they are important for the ethics of practice. It is also the case that public opinion is affected by the high-profile cases.

Unintended consequences of reports and government responses and initiatives mean that there is a danger of them becoming part of the problem rather than the solution. Government response focuses public attention: for example, David Cameron's (Prime Minister of the day) suggestion that nurses should make hourly rounds of patients to avoid problems such as the one precipitating the 999 call. Hourly rounds may or may not be a good idea, it depends upon the setting. However all that may be, the qualification for making suggestions as to how to go about nursing does not reside in the leader of the government.

Legitimate criticism has its place, but when the media line up all the problems that are hitting the headlines, sometimes not making clear the difference between criminal negligence and problems that stem from organisational shortcomings, funding and staffing shortages, the picture of a profession and service in crisis is portrayed – they are, of course, focussing on *their* job of selling news. Sociological analysis would tell us that this is not a representative picture of the NHS: importantly this misleading image does damage in terms of recruitment and retention. Whilst no one has an interest in keeping nurses in the profession who are not performing to the professional and ethical standards, the wider picture of the professional image has to be kept in mind.

---

[8]Beverly Allitt was found guilty of murdering four children in 1991, and attempting the murder of three others and causing grievous bodily harm to six children; she was imprisoned for 30 years.

At the same time that the press reports and government suggestions were coming out, there was a report from the Royal College of Nursing (RCN) proposing staff:patient ratios that they maintain would make for safe care (RCN, 2012). Evidence in the form of a RCN survey (2010) of 1,700 nurses was also produced. This survey reported (on the basis of the most recent duty they worked) that 78 per cent of nurses said that they were unable to comfort or talk with patients adequately because of low staffing numbers. Also, 34 per cent of nurses said they had not enough time for helping with feeding patients, and a similar percentage had not sufficient time to assist with patients getting to the toilet and managing incontinence. This is just a small snapshot at a particular time, so little can be made of it here. It is included to demonstrate that the research data that social and statistical research can provide gives us the wider picture and demonstrates how complex the matter of getting care right is. Given this picture, a concern with smiling seems rather superficial. Working with insufficient staff or poor use of available staff is difficult enough, but against a background of criticism from the media there are wider concerns.

The RCN suggested more practical responses, calling for a staff to patient ratio ratio of 1:7 (at the time of writing it is around 1:9). The RCN report their members as saying that there are too few qualified staff on duty and because of this they claim that there is not enough time to help with feeding of patients or with attending to their hygiene needs. The problem is made worse by the media attention and negative public opinion, in spite of which the work has to go on and so nurses have to go on. All of this adds to the complexity of the context in which nursing care takes place. Nursing is at times a stressful occupation, and this press attention and general criticism of the whole profession only exacerbates the stress.

Under the Labour government there was the Prime Minister's Commission on the Future of Nursing and Midwifery in England where, among other things, the big idea was to have the *nurses' pledge*:

> This was a pledge to deliver high quality care. Nurses and midwives must renew their pledge to society and service users to tackle unacceptable variations in standards and deliver high quality, compassionate care. (Prime Minister's Commission, 2010: taken from the 20 'high-level recommendations' of the report)

The idea of a pledge was in response to a series of problems in both acute hospitals and care homes where the practice fell far short of the standards required by both the NMC *Code of Professional Conduct* (2008) and the legal requirements set for care facilities. The pledge may have played well to the public, but in professional terms it was not seen to offer much beyond the level of gesture. After the change of government at the next election the fact that it was a Prime Minister's Commission made it the 'wrong Prime Minister' and the Commission's Report, which did contain some useful commentary, was lost in the zeal of the incoming government plans. The new Prime Minister was not slow in getting involved with the NHS, and there were photo-opportunities and press calls with the Prime Minister displaying his knowledge of the hospital infection control (MRSA and C. *difficile*) and following the dress rules – no necktie and sleeves rolled up to the elbow. If the solution really were a pledge and the mass introduction of an hourly ward round, there would be little problem. These politicians' 'solutions' can be double-edged swords, welcomed by some as a good thing that politicians take an interest, but resented by others who see it as interference in what are professional concerns. Whatever the profession's view of individual initiatives, inquiries and campaigns, the spotlight being on nursing is a mixed blessing.

Workforce planning and arriving at the optimum staffing levels for clinical staff have to be understood in a wider context of recruitment and student numbers set alongside the expected number of retirals. Other factors which affect the quality of care include the throughput of patients and the numbers of admissions. The politicians' view of an increase in patient throughput in a hospital is different from a clinical view. In political success terms, more patients treated and admitted represents good and efficient use of resources. However, from a clinical perspective admitting more patients for shorter stays puts pressure on the staff and the infection control measures are less effective: full occupancy is not good for infection rates. This is an organisational fact of running the service; it does not excuse poor care but it does highlight the fact that the complexity of the system has to be taken into account when change is planned.

Nursing is notoriously difficult to define. Despite the volume of literature on nursing theory and such, we often return to the 'what is nursing?' question. Meantime the public image of nursing has a higher profile than do the profession's own perceptions and ambitions.

If I were to hazard a working definition of nursing it would lean heavily on that provided by Virginia Henderson (1964) back in the early 1960s, when she stated that nursing was essentially doing for patients that which they cannot do for themselves. The fact that this definition is nearly half a century old is of no matter because the core of nursing has not changed. Advances in technology, the developments in medical science, especially in genetics and pharmacology, and the social change that has taken place since Henderson defined nursing have brought about a radically different health service. There remains at its centre a relationship based on trust. Trust between professional and patient. Relationships between nurse and patient, between doctor and patient and between patients and a number of other clinical practitioners are all based on professionalism and trust. It is within this context of trusting relationships that health care is effected. One of the interests, then, in looking at the organisational context within which health care takes place is to see how this trust is produced and sustained.

Teamwork in Health Care

Teamwork relies upon the different disciplines coming together with different skills and knowledge to achieve the common goal of patient care. Teams are only as strong as their constituent parts; for multi-disciplinary teamwork to be successful, the professions involved have to be prepared to work in different ways and not to retreat to their professional hinterlands when the going gets rough. The give and take required for health care professionals to arrive at moral consensus on difficult

decisions is also required for effective teamwork in clinical practice, hence my asser-
tion that if you can do teamwork, you can do ethics (Melia, 2004).

One aim of my study of health care ethics in intensive care was to bring together
the sociological analysis of how the care is actually brought about and the moral
philosophical perspective on what that care *should* entail. We have seen that ethics
for nursing practice is concerned with moral debates and draw upon the arguments
and theories of moral philosophers. A sociological analysis is helpful in allowing us
to get a handle on how the health care professionals engage in and act upon these
moral principles. The main focus of the study was upon the sociological analysis of
clinical practice, which allowed an examination of the social organisation of that
practice. It provided an analysis of the context within which ethical issues arise and
must be handled. The context is sometimes part of the problem and, of necessity, has
to be considered in its resolution.

A similar work concerned with sociology and ethics is that of Zussman (1992). His
concern was with medical ethics, particularly with informed consent and decisions
to withdraw treatment in the intensive care unit (ICU). He argued for the sociological analysis because medical ethics tends to concentrate on how decisions *should* be
made and so misses out on how they *are* made in daily practice. Sociological empirical work is important in gaining this understanding of how decisions are made.

In fact, Zussman set out to write about medical ethics. His study is about, in his
words:

> informed consent, the limitation of potentially life-prolonging treatment, and the
> allocation of scarce resources in two intensive care units. (1992: 1)

Zussman says that his book is not a work of medical ethics, which he says addresses
matters of right and wrong. To these matters he said there was little to add from his
study; instead he described his book as being about:

> the ways in which right and wrong are interpreted and used – about the ways in
> which conceptions of right and wrong emerge out of social situations of patients
> and their families, doctors and nurses from the workings of hospitals and the courts.
> (1992: 1)

This encapsulates the way in which ethics for practice works, and demonstrates the
role that sociological analysis can play in this.

In the study of ethics in intensive care there was a lot of discussion about team
work and the power relationships between the members of the team (Melia, 2004).
The social practices involved in the day-to-day organisation of health care, when
examined through the methods of sociology, demonstrate how the team brings about
care and treatment. The experience of teamwork allows the different members of the
health care team to air their opinions and to discuss the moral aspects of a case and
so to work together in a kind of ethical teamwork. The practice of teamwork exer-
cises the communication and understanding 'muscles' needed for ethical discussion
and the resolution of the ethical questions which have come to be associated with
health care. One of the main conclusions was that:

In a very general sense there is no hierarchy in the moral positions taken by members of the team. The balance of ethical analysis does not depend upon the technical or scientific expertise possessed by the holder of a particular moral view. All opinions on the team carry equal weight in a moral sense; it is the social processes which promote consensus that are important to the smooth running of the ICU. (Melia, 2004: 137)

This extract makes plain that the social context of care is an important factor in the quality of the care. Also it is worth noting in passing that it was a sociological analysis that led to these conclusions. The 'lessons from intensive care' (Melia, 2004) were, as the book's sub-title suggests, lessons applicable more widely to health care. One of the important lessons for the smooth functioning of teams, both within and across disciplines, is that they should know how to disagree and continue to function as a team. Knowing how to do this is the key to getting through the difficult moral terrain of health care.

The political climate in which the health service is operating has an effect on the service and the morale of the staff. Health is invariably one of the important issues in an election and politicians have the life of a parliament in which to achieve their ambitions for health; this tends to produce a rather short-term approach to targets and goals in health. The professionals in health care are in it for the longer haul, and this gives rise to conflict between the clinicians and those holding the purse strings. These differences manifest themselves in various ways, an important one being the allocation of resources. There are occasions where it is argued that clinical decisions are being made by health service managers rather than the clinicians. Waiting times for surgery and discharge policies are areas of concern in this respect (Syal, 2013).

Sociological analysis of some of the ethical issues encountered in health care brings an understanding of the practical workings of nursing ethics. The combination of both sociological and philosophical perspectives assists in our understanding of the moral dimension of health care practice, because the social organisation of health care practice is an important part of the social context of care. Changes in the organisation of health care have their impact on those working in health care. The clinical and social context in which ethical questions about practice are addressed is important if we are to take account of the working practices and professional cultures of those involved. How a society provides for the social and health care of its older members is a central question for 21st-century health care.

- The clinical and social context in which ethical questions about practice are addressed is important.
- Aristotle thought that ethics is a practical matter and relates to practical situations.
- If you can do teamwork you can do ethics.
- The combination of both sociological and philosophical perspectives assists in our understanding of the moral dimension of health care practice.

4

Individual Conscience
Approach to Ethics

The heart has its reasons which reason knows nothing of.

Blaise Pascal, 1670

This chapter takes as its point of departure a focus on the role of the individual's conscience in determining what is right and wrong in our own actions and those of others. In a broader philosophical sense we are talking about how we decide what is right and wrong and how to behave in accordance with that judgement. In the context of this book, we are concerned with rights and wrongs in relation to nursing practice. As we have said, ethics is not about dictating what is right and wrong, rather it seeks to examine how individuals work out what is right and wrong and how they act on this and make decisions when moral questions are involved.

The debates about the rights and wrongs of health care can be discussed by reference to four main principles: beneficence and non-maleficence, respect for persons (autonomy) and justice (see Chapter 2). In considering the patient's best interests, the idea of harm versus good is theoretically a good starting point. Indeed it is also a good practical starting point. There is, though, the question of how do we know what the right thing to do is? How do we decide what is right? The question is probably more philosophical than practical, however it demands a response which can be acted upon.

The distinction between practical and theoretical reasoning is relevant here. This distinction has it that *practical reason* is designed for action and *theoretical reasoning* leads to knowledge that we can accept on the basis of reason. Practical reasoning is our main interest in this book, with a view to examining the nature of the thinking that lies behind the business of making decisions in patient care.

A staff nurse arrives on a busy ward in the morning to take charge of the first shift of the day. She is feeling tired following a birthday celebration the previous evening. She is responsible for organising, among many other things, the meal breaks across the 12-hour shift. There are a number of complex matters to be raised with the senior medical staff and there is an IT consultant due to assist with a problem with the computers. The charge nurse is due to work through the afternoon and early evening. The staff nurse knows that by convention she should take her breaks early before all this activity begins so that she can co-ordinate the work and cover the breaks for others. However, there is a very attractive option of waiting until mid-morning for her break and then taking a late lunch to coincide with the second peak in the day's activity.

This is not a moral dilemma by any means, but it is an example of moral choice. The situation described is one in which the staff nurse has an opportunity to consider other's needs ahead of her own. The staff nurse does not need anyone's permission to take advantage of this situation to suit her own needs. The ward and patients would be better served if she organised not to be away at the busy points, but it would not be causing any clear harm. The unknowns in the situation cannot be brought into the equation, the 'what if' this or that happened when she was absent from the ward. Others are capable of managing, and in any case things can go wrong when the senior staff are off the ward for good reasons as well as bad. So why is this even worth thinking about? It will be a matter for individual opinion – more properly individual conscience – to come to a view on this. Is there a right thing to do? If so, why, and what makes it right? Would suiting her own needs be wrong, or just not as right?

Individual Conscience

One way of looking at how we go about working out how to act for the good of the patient is to consider how ethical theories might offer some guide to practice. Ethical theory is a useful resource that stands a little removed from the individual conscience. A useful approach to thinking about this, offered by Campbell (1984), is to start with a consideration of the subjective workings of individual conscience and move from there along the continuum leading towards more objectivity. So, to anticipate here some of the content of later chapters, we start out by considering the individual conscience, which is essentially a rather private view, and proceed to consider increasingly more objective theories along what might be thought of as a continuum with subjectivity and objectivity at its opposing ends. This includes utilitarian ideas of the greatest benefit for the greatest number, duty-based ethics, rights-based approaches and virtue ethics, where the nature of the practitioner is central to the theory.

When thinking about the treatment of patients, nurses are often encouraged to ask themselves 'how would this be if it were my mother?'. This is quite an individual approach to the question. On the other hand, the moment we start to think of what is possible for patients, there enters a question of fairness, of wanting to treat all patients alike; that is, a desire to do the best for everyone. There is an objectivity about this approach, an approach which, as we see in Chapter 7, can be described as utilitarian – the greatest good for the greatest number. Within this idea come issues of equality, fair dealing and justice.

But for the present, let us stay with the individual conscience. Conscience is, of course, not entirely private and anyone who has a faith, or has experienced the influence that a faith has on others, will have been exposed to discussion of the nature of conscience. Whilst conscience is essentially a private business, the idea of conscience is a public matter and one that is referred to in everyday life. A conscience is not a secret, everyone knows what is meant by conscience; what is less knowable is how it operates and how to justify what it comes up with. Politicians talk of doing the right thing. We speak of moral standards, and changes in the nature of society are often couched in terms of different, usually lower, standards of public behaviour. Such comments can be a generalised expression of things not being what they used to be. It may also be a generational-led complaint about the activities of a profession, that things were somehow better in the rose-tinted vision of the past.

Nursing has been attacked in various ways in the wake of genuine failures of care.[1] Sometimes the attack is more vague, where usually one generation of nurses accuses the next of being less able, less compassionate, less kind or caring than previous generations were. The complaints are not always easily substantiated and are sometimes more to do with perception than reality. In expressing views on morality or other societal debates people will sometimes preface their comments with the caveat that they speak as a Christian, Muslim, Jew or any other persuasion, before going on to express the view they hold. Those of a different religious persuasion, or of none, may interpret such a statement from a different perspective from that of the speaker. Or they might agree with the view and regard it as right and proper and moral, and not see what a religious faith has to do with it. By and large, the particularities of the perspectives of different faiths are not to the point in these situations; rather it is the basic values that underlie the expression of the rights and wrongs of the matter that count. At one level, it matters more that nurses provide the necessary assistance to ensure that a patient receives sufficient food and drink and be properly nourished than it does to know upon what belief system, if any, the nursing care rests. At another level, it is clearly better if the professional care of patients is based on more than technical knowledge and competence. The motivation to care cannot be taught without some consideration of the ethical basis for practice.

The individual conscience approach to ethics assumes that people have some inbuilt means of knowing what is right and wrong. The inner voice that we know

---

[1]Report of the Mid Staffordshire NHS Foundation Trust Public Inquiry (Francis, 2013) being not the only case, but it is a particularly stark example.

as 'conscience' works within the wider societal idea of what is right and wrong, what is acceptable or not. There is an understandable attraction to the more 'objective' approaches because a move away from individual conscience makes societal debate and professional ethics more feasible. Campbell puts it well when he says of what he calls 'the *plain man's* feeling that his [*sic*] conscience knows best' approach:

> [W]e might say that such a view seems sensible enough until we meet two plain men who disagree. (1984: 36)

This is a very good point and so easily allows us to regard the gendered language that Campbell uses merely as a product of its time.

Moral Choice

Ethics is concerned with studying the morality or moral values upon which groups of people and societies base their actions. The moral positions which people adopt and the values they hold tend to be personal and intuitive. That is not to say that they are individualistic in an anarchic sense – groups of people will hold similar values and in that sense they are more than one person's view. Nevertheless, the values that we as individuals hold do tend to be rather more intuitive than objective and as such not readily defended in the face of alternatives which other consciences might produce. It is important to recognise that when we move beyond the individual and into the social or professional realm, the moral positions that we adopt have to be reasoned and argued for and not merely asserted. The kinds of arguments made to justify our moral positions will vary, although in general they can be said to be, to greater and lesser extents, objective: objective in the sense that they go beyond the personal and can be explained to others without any pre-requisites of opinion, belief or faith. The moral reason for making one choice over another has to do with what is regarded as right, or perhaps at least not wrong. It is important to note that this is not a question of being either subjective or objective, it is more a question of balance, somewhere between the two. So long as there is a move away from the idea that private, individual conscience is all that matters we will be getting somewhere in terms of objectivity and having regard for the views and values of others.

This chapter is about moving from an individual view of right and wrong to something more objective, something that can be signed up to, as it were, by a wider society. Philosophers have over the years built up bodies of work, abstract models, conveying a sense of how society should be: how we should act as a group, society, as individuals within society and for the good of that society. When we carry this idea over into health care we find nurses and other health care professionals working out how to deliver care in a fair and just way with the interests of the patient being paramount. The formalised manifestation of these ambitions for good ethical care comes in the form of professional codes of conduct (more on codes of conduct in Chapter 9). These documents state the principles that underlie practice. The translation of these ideals into practice depends upon the individual professionals and upon the context in which they work.

In other words, the mere statement of ideals, how things ought to be, will not in itself bring about the desired results in terms of practice.

Socrates and Aristotle and other ancient Greek philosophers were interested in the question of how to lead a good life – good for the individual and for society. Even the most scant knowledge of history would tell us that there is at least a part of human nature which is driven to war, to acts of destruction and to violence, which make the idea of always acting in ways conducive to a good life somewhat fanciful. Yet we can also see acts of humanity, generosity and kindness throughout history and around us now which give hope. Human beings are clearly complex and their motives for action equally so. In attempting to understand the ways in which nursing as a profession sets about caring for people in ways which can be said to be ethical, we need to acknowledge that nurses are themselves members of society and are therefore as prone to both good and bad behaviour as the next person. However, as nurses, individuals have to behave according to professional standards, which are enshrined in a code of ethical conduct. Individual behaviour will always depend, to a degree, upon individual values and an individual's capacity for trustworthy action, and so there is a need to move towards a more objective view of rights and wrongs when it comes to professional behaviour.

In making the move from individual conscience-based ideas about ethics to a more objective approach it is standard practice in text books of this kind to turn to those moral philosophers who take a less individualistic approach to moral questions. A common way to move from individual conscience theories to something more objective is to look to Kant's work on universal imperatives or the utilitarian writings of Bentham and Mill, or to consider rights-based ethics. More of these in later chapters. Suffice it to say here that these are ethical theories which address the moral questions that arise in practice by appealing to reason and general principles which can be expressed and shared without recourse to an individual conscience or to a faith or belief system.

However, before moving to these approaches it is worth taking a look at how we move from the individual conscience approach to something with a wider base. It helps to be able to point to more widely held social values when attempting to justify our moral position on, for instance, decision making in relation to end-of-life care. The wider basis for our view takes us a step away from the sole reference point of our own individual conscience. Most people if asked about what they would do when they are in a situation where there is a moral decision to be made are likely to make some reference to the idea of a conscience. The idea of a conscience is frequently reinforced by belief in a divine being, giving some backing, as it were, to the moral principles that are attached to the individual conscience. Even those with no particular religious belief may still invest their conscience with some importance in terms of a generalised view of human decency (for a fuller discussion, see Campbell, 1984).

Natural and Divine Law

Even when we when we try to move from individual conscience to the idea of a natural law, we find that there are long-standing links between the two. The ancient Greek philosophers thought that natural law was there to be found and that man was part of it and it was up to man to determine their place in this natural order. Campbell best sums up the difficulty here when he says:

> Fundamental to the concept of natural law is the distinction between natural and unnatural, which in turn depends on the view that all things serve a certain end or purpose. Natural law is regarded as that which delineates the true, or divinely intended end of man. (1984: 69)

To take an example, abortion is regarded by some to be against divine will and is in that way unnatural and so cannot be considered part of the natural law within which mankind needs to find a way of living within the natural order. This idea of finding our place in the natural order of the world, as we have seen, goes back all the way to Aristotle (see Chapter 1). This alone gives us some idea of the appeal, and perhaps the weight, that natural law has for us as human beings. But if we are looking to include those who do not have a belief in a deity, then this circularity between divine and natural law reasoning is a problem. Without making light of it, the problem is akin to the explanation for a two-year-old as to why they should do this or that 'because I say so' will not do for an answer. In a heterogeneous and secular society to say 'because God says so' is not going to do either, not least because we arrive back at the question 'How do we know?'. Whether the question is 'How do we know it is right?' or 'How do we know that God said it was right?', the question remains 'How do we know?'. Justification for the morality of a decision is the point at issue and the terrain of moral philosophy.

The idea of a natural law, one which human beings will follow without divine direction, has its appeal. The various writings and discussions of the right thing to do invariably lead to the idea of the laws of nature. It is useful to turn to natural law theory and see what this has to offer in the quest for answers to the question 'How do we know what is the right thing to do in particular circumstances?'. The linkage between natural and unnatural goes further, and in some theological writings the link is clear where the natural is defined as good and the unnatural as evil. The crux of the problem here is well described by Campbell (1984: see Ch.4 for full discussion). On this analysis, whereby natural law and divine revelation are linked, God is seen as the ultimate word when it comes to good and evil. The expectation is that people should use their reasoning powers to work out the difference between what is good and what is evil. In doing this they arrive at the same conclusion as the one to be found in divine law. Campbell sums this up neatly when he says:

> Such an account of natural law appears to see faith and rationality as two independent streams flowing from the same source, without contamination, as it were, of the one by the other. (1984: 71)

Aristotle's answer to the question of how we should live is that we should fit in with the natural law. Campbell et al. note that:

> Aquinas and some of the Christian Moralists have grafted onto Aristotle's theory the doctrine that the ideal of human function is the way we are meant to be because it represents the design of our Creator. This, like the Aristotelian tradition, allows us to examine what counts as human excellence or well-being in an attempt to discover how we should act. Aristotle's view is, however, consistent with an underlying theory about human nature and its origins, including an evolutionary one. (2005: 3)

With or without the involvement of a deity or faith in the workings of a conscience it is generally held that some sort of sense of right and wrong resides in us as human beings. It is perhaps comforting to think this, but how do we know that a conscience is working well, and how do we determine what working well means? When we consider the incidents, which come about every so often, that lead to inquiries and reports detailing poor care and sometimes downright cruel behaviour in hospitals and care homes, we have to question the workings of individual conscience.

Natural law is not so straightforward as it may seem. The idea, as old as Aristotle, is that there is order, and that we, as human beings with the power of reason, are capable of working out how we should function within that natural law, and function for the common good.

> What is right for us to do and what is good for us to do are matters that do depend on and refer back to our common human nature. To that extent there is 'natural law'. (MacCormick, 2008: 200)

The link between the revelation of divine law and natural law is often somewhat vague. Here is not the place for a theological discussion. However, if we can judge our behaviour and that of others against some norm, we must reasonably ask how we come by these generalised rules for moral behaviour. In other words, how do we arrive at these natural laws? To shed light on this I draw on MacCormick's work. As a lawyer and philosopher he is not primarily concerned with theology, but with the philosophy of law, with justice and with the question 'Can reason be practical?'. This question is for the legal profession, and it is concerned with making the link between the principles underlying the law and the business of making it work in practice. How do we know that what we are doing is in keeping with the underlying principles? In that sense MacCormick is asking about the way we work out what to do and how we know that we have chosen the right thing. This is a practical question and one that we can recognise in nursing. The judgements here are clinical but the situation is practical and the questions in part moral. Practical reason is in this sense as important for nursing practice as it is for the practice of law.

In the context of a discussion of the extent to which moral autonomy can be an individual matter, MacCormick explains that we can reconcile individual autonomy and the existence of faith and religion if we accept that human beings are:

creatures of God, taking their place in the natural, evolved and still evolving universe, a universe which is entirely in God's creation, then humans have the psychology they have because they acquired it through a Divinely initiated evolutionary process. (2008: 95–6)

This kind of thinking is very different from the philosophers who seek to explain moral behaviour without recourse to a deity or belief. MacCormick (2008: 57) notes that Adam Smith and David Hume sought to root the understanding of morality in a naturalistic account of human passions and sentiments.

Hume was an atheist (Priest, 1990: 161) and thought that reason and emotion played a part in the discussion of moral questions. Hume famously said that:

[r]eason is, and ought only to be, the slave of the passions, and can never pretend to any other office than to serve and obey them. ([1777] 1978: 415)

In making this statement he clearly believes that the way in which we reason and think things through in order to understand the world and our place within it includes the passions: in other words, the way in which we reason must include the emotional part of our nature.

David Hume was a leading philosopher of the 18th-century Enlightenment. The Enlightenment was a period in which the scientific approach to knowledge took hold and changed for ever the way in which we regard knowledge and what counts as proof or evidence of knowledge. Hume's influence on philosophy stems from, among other things, the rejection of the drawing upon the knowledge of divine law or values that come from outside of the human experience. Hume's views stood out in stark contrast to those which historically had prevailed. These ideas held that the natural order of things could be arrived at through reason and thinking. Hume would not cause a stir today on this count because we expect ideas to have some basis in evidence or observation. But in Hume's day it was acceptable to reason one's way to theory by way of logic and mathematics. Hume's empiricism (i.e. basing knowledge on data from observation or experience) is the approach of science. The essence of the method is that knowledge is based on observable facts. In Hume's (1777 [1978: 415]) words, 'nothing is in the mind that was not first in the senses', an 18th-century way of saying that if one cannot evidence it from experience, it cannot be said to exist.

Moral Sentiments (Emotions)

In this chapter we consider Adam Smith's work. His ideas offer a means of moving away from a subjective approach to ethics. Smith (1723–90) was a scholar of the 18th-century Enlightenment and following his friend and fellow philosopher, David Hume (1711–76), sought to write philosophy without relying on divine law or religious belief. Smith is remembered mainly for his important contribution to economics through his book *The Wealth of Nations* ([1776] 1999). But Smith was also a philosopher and it is his work *The Theory of Moral Sentiments* ([1790] 2009) that is of interest here. Smith's idea, put very briefly, was that we need to be aware of the part that human sentiments play in arriving at judgements about right and wrong. MacCormick points out that the more contemporary term would be 'empathy'. It is interesting to note too, that whilst it is his book *The Wealth of Nations* with which we tend to associate him, Smith produced no fewer than six editions of the *Theory of Moral Sentiments* from 1759 with the most substantially revised 6th edition being published shortly before his death in 1790. This is of note because, whilst others might have seen the two main themes of his books as separate endeavours, for Smith there existed links between the two works. This is described by Sen (in Smith, [1790] 2009: Introduction), who says that whilst Smith himself drew upon his *Theory of Moral Sentiments* in the production of *The Wealth of Nations*, it was largely ignored by others throughout the 19th and 20th centuries and he was mostly known for his contribution to economics. The consequence of this was, as Sen puts it, that:

> the typical understanding of the *Wealth of Nations* has been constrained, to the detriment of economics as a subject. (Sen, in Smith, [1790] 2009: Introduction)

Sen goes on to note that there are further consequences of that neglect. These remarks are especially pertinent in the light of the world economic recession, which started with the banking crisis of 2008. Sen says that the neglect of Smith's *The Theory of Moral Sentiments* applies to:

> the need for recognizing the plurality of human motivations, the connections between ethics and economics, and the co-dependent – rather than free-standing – role of institutions in general and free markets in particular in the functioning of the economy. (Sen, in Smith, [1790] 2009: viii)

Sen (in Smith, [1790] 2009) describes the intentions of Smith, which he says some economists of the day missed and some have continued to miss in the 21st century. The idea that self-interest is the motivation for markets stuck, and this explains, according to Sen, why there are still different interpretations of Adam Smith's work. Nevertheless, the fact that we are still discussing his work and finding it relevant more than 250 years since its publication is testament to the relevance of its message. One reading of Smith's *The Wealth of Nations* suggests that self-interest will pay. The so-called 'rational choice' theory dictates that the rational way to behave in economics is to follow an essentially selfish (Smith would say 'self-love') policy in order to be economically successful. Sen (in Smith, [1790] 2009: x) points out that this was to misunderstand because Smith, with his idea of self-love as motivation, was referring to the exchange part of the economy and the motivation for exchange. He was not referring to other important parts of the economic system, namely production and distribution. Smith discussed other motives, beyond self-interest, which also helps the market and the functioning of the economy. These other motives included humanity, justice, generosity and public spirit.[2] These motives, it seems to me, would suit nursing practice just as well as Smith thought them relevant to the market economy.

Sen's point is that rather than regarding Smith's work as two separate entities, sentiments and money, it is closer to his intentions to see that there are links between his *Theory of Moral Sentiments* and *The Wealth of Nations*. Of the six editions he published of *The Theory Moral Sentiments*,[3] four came before and two after the publication of his book *The Wealth of Nations*. So we can think of *The Wealth of Nations* as being wrapped around, as it were, by the ideas that Smith was developing from edition to edition of *The Theory of Moral Sentiments*. Adam Smith's ideas in the book that the economists seized upon were very much influenced by his thinking about the part that emotions ('sentiment', in his words) play in the motivations that are at work in market economies. These links can be seen, for example, in his discussion of a wide range of motivations which play a part in people's engagement with the economy, motivations which go beyond self-love, or self-interest as we would have it today.

With his theory of moral sentiments Smith was to break away from the ways in which philosophers worked at the time, ways which followed the established pattern of working of the moral philosophers in the ancient Greek tradition: that is, through an abstract approach to the study of morals. The abstract approach was not removed from the practical matters in life because the theoretical discussions were applied to the practical questions of the day, questions about how to live a good life. The move from the abstract principles of philosophical argument to a more human approach was essentially what the 18th-century philosophers David Hume and Adam Smith were about. They discussed morality from the basis of a very human account of how we behave towards one another.

Impartial Spectator

In Smith's opening words to *The Theory of Moral Sentiments* he says:

> How selfish soever man may be supposed, there are evidently some principles in his nature, which interest him in the fortune of others, and render their happiness necessary to him, though he derives nothing from it except the pleasure of seeing it. ([1790] 2009)

---

[2]For further discussion see Sen's Introduction in Smith ([1790] 2009).

[3]Smith published six editions of *Theory of Moral Sentiments* between 1759 and 1790, with the last in the year of his death.

Smith goes on to say:

> That we often derive sorrow from the sorrow of others, is a matter of fact too obvi-ous to require any instances to prove it; for this sentiment, like all the other original passions of human nature, is by no means confined to the virtuous and humane, though they perhaps may feel it with the most exquisite sensibility. The greatest ruffian, the most hardened violator of the laws of society, is not altogether without it. ([1790] 2009: 13)

In fact, MacCormick (2008: 57) says that Adam Smith's work *The Theory of Moral Sentiments* makes a good place to look for less abstract approaches to ethics. The reason lies in the fact that Smith takes a very practical approach to his study of the interactions of human beings. Smith says that as humans we are capable of reacting to the experiences of others – the automatic wince when we witness someone trip and fall, or bang their head on a shelf as they stand up, or knock their shin on a table leg as they sit down. This reaction that we have to the experiences of others, Smith says, demonstrates our capacity to feel for others.

Hume and Smith argued that human beings are capable of sympathy. Smith says that the human capacity to 'feel' for others, in both their fortunes and misfortunes, is the basis of our capacity for moral judgement. This capacity extends both to our own actions and those of others. This idea of observing oneself, as it were, and judg-ing one's own behaviour is described by Smith in terms of what he calls an 'impartial spectator'. Put briefly, this idea of the 'impartial spectator' is that we can think of an imaginary person whom we can run our ideas by, as it were, to check if we are thinking along the same lines as other right-minded people might think. The idea is that we can step aside from ourselves and attempt to view our actions and plans from the perspective of another, a more impartial other. It is a way of bringing some objectivity to the workings of our individual conscience.

This lengthy quotation from Smith's work makes the point in his own words:

> The principle by which we naturally either approve or disapprove of our own con-duct, seems to be altogether the same with that by which we exercise the like judgements concerning the conduct of other people. We either approve or disap-prove of the conduct of another man according as we feel that, when we bring his case home to ourselves, we either can or cannot entirely sympathize with the sentiments and motives which directed it. And, in the same manner, we either approve or disapprove of our own conduct, as we feel that, when we place our-selves in the situation of another man, and view it, as it were, with his eyes and from his station, we either can or cannot entirely enter into and sympathize with the sentiments and motives which influenced it. We can never survey our own sen-timents and motives, we can never form any judgement concerning them, unless we remove ourselves, as it were, from our own natural station and endeavour to view them as at a certain distance from us. But we can do this in no other way than by endeavouring to view them with the eyes of other people, or as other people are likely to view. ([1790] 2009: 133)

Smith goes on to say:

> We endeavour to examine our own conduct as we imagine any other fair and impartial spectator would examine it. If, upon placing ourselves in his situation, we thoroughly enter into all the passions and motives which influenced it, we approve of it, by sympathy with the approbation of this supposed equitable judge. If otherwise, we enter into his disapprobation, and condemn it. ([1790] 2009: 133)

MacCormick explains how this 'impartial spectator' notion works by describing graphically the difference in feelings of the affected and those of the more 'impartial spectator'. He says:

> An incident that has annoyed you, who were the target of the malevolence, arouses sympathetic anger in me, not blind rage. This is a fact of which all human beings come to be aware. (2008: 57–8)

In clinical practice, deciding whether or not to report an error or omission in care is a matter of individual moral judgement. If no one other than the person concerned is aware of the omission, it is already a matter of moral judgement.

> For example, if a nurse fails to administer a treatment or to give medications at the correct time provided that no harm is done it might go unreported if the nurse concerned sees no wrong-doing in the situation. In plain language, less fuss would ensue if no reporting takes place.

This 'least said, soonest mended' approach might appear to be a common-sense response, but the wider ramifications of such behaviour in an organisation carry consequences, moral and practical. The idea of an 'impartial spectator', someone removed from a situation, and therefore less subjective, is a point of reference, something against which to judge oneself. MacCormick says that the 'impartial spectator' idea enables people to 'normalize or even rationalize their emotional responses in mutual interaction' (2008: 1–2). In the example of the medication error, had a colleague been there to witness the omission then the nurse might have behaved differently, or asked the colleague's opinion. The 'impartial spectator' is an impartial source of a second opinion.

In some ways recourse to the idea of an 'impartial spectator' is not dissimilar to the idea of asking yourself whether you would do this if no one were looking. It is essentially Plato's question, 'Would we be good if we knew that there would be no consequences of our actions?'. The distressing postings of personal remarks and other negative comments on someone's life that can be found on the Internet and so-called social networking sites are some kind of evidence of what people will do if they think that no one knows who they are. This would suggest that there is some heed paid to social sanction and the generalised sense of a standard of behaviour to which we should adhere.

Impartiality – Reason – Emotion

Smith's idea of the 'impartial spectator' was to gain some external view of one's actions and motives. To an extent the spectator was a way of validating or justifying one's actions by the knowledge that it is what others would do. 'Impartial spectator' reasoning is a way to validate that inner conscience, inner voice, instinct, call it what you will, to show that others do much the same thing. We have noted that there is a desire among moral theorists to move away from the subjective view of morality of the individual conscience theories. Adam Smith's 'impartial spectator' is a rather different way of moving away from the subjective individual conscience approach to ethics. Smith was interested in looking for objectivity and spoke of impartiality and universality. Smith thought that it is our capacity to judge ourselves and to judge others that forms the basis of our moral reason.

The full title of Hume's, work generally known as *A Treatise of Human Nature* (first published in 1739), is *A Treatise of Human Nature: Being an Attempt to Introduce the Experimental Method of Reasoning into Moral Subjects*. In writing this book Hume was conveying his ideas about the passions and free will. Hume also wrote about some of the moral debates that we are concerned with here, namely justice, beneficence and obligation. Hume departed from the usual style of philosophical writing and introduced, as the full title of the book states, what he called the 'experimental method of reasoning'. By this he did not mean experiment as we would understand it today – he was referring to 'experience'. The idea was to explain the world in terms of what could be observed or experienced; we would now refer to this as empirical work, which would be based on data. Smith did not seek to be entirely analytic and rational (in the sense of applying reason) in his 'impartial spectator' approach to deciding upon the rights and wrongs of human actions. He believed that the moral sentiments should enter into the equation when it came to deciding upon the right way to act.

As we are talking about being sympathetic to the plight of others it follows that the emotional aspect of our nature must figure in the judgements that we make. Campbell says that:

> our approval of the pleasure of another is based on our ability to share in his experience as though it were our own. (1984: 111)

Campbell goes on to describe Hume's approach to this sympathetic view of the experiences of others:

> Hume sees no opposition between self-interest and benevolence, and no need to reduce one to the other. Anything which serves the common cause of humanity will naturally be approved by all reasonable men. (1984: 111)

Campbell continues with a brief quotation from Hume, which he says is worth including for 'its entertaining polemic style'; on the same grounds, especially for the style, I include it here. Campbell explains that Hume spoke of having no time for what the Enlightenment philosopher called 'a whole train of monkish virtues', by which he meant celibacy, fasting, humility and the like. Hume discussed these as 'vices' since he thought that they were neither useful nor enjoyable, and he dismissed those possessing these virtues/vices, saying:

> A gloomy hare-brained enthusiast, after his death, may have a place in the calendar; but will scarcely ever be admitted, when alive, into intimacy and society, except by those who are as delirious and dismal as himself. (Hume, ([1777] 1902), in Campbell, 1984: 111–12)

Campbell et al. (2005: 3) say that we can see similarities and connections between Aristotle's work and that of Hume, and in their discussion of medical ethics they take what they describe as a 'leap from Aristotle to David Hume' in order to take us to 'the naturalistic theory' of Hume. The leap from Aristotle's idea of what constitutes the good life is a leap to Hume's idea, which is:

> the form that constitutes right living is taken to be exemplified by decent, clear-thinking, eighteenth-century gentlemen. (Campbell et al., 2005: 3)

The fact that a sensible leap can be taken from Aristotle, the 4th-century BC Greek philosopher, to the 18th-century philosopher of the Scottish Enlightenment is testament to the robust nature of the ideas of the early philosophers when it comes to ethics. Times and context have changed, but the fundamental questions and some of their answers remain the same.

MacCormick (2008: 5–9) says that we are not naturally impartial and that unless we can actually ask advice of an impartial person we must, as he puts it, 'cultivate a capacity for abstraction from our own partisan involvement'.

MacCormick also notes that Smith's idea of the 'impartial spectator' sits well with the psychology of human beings, as we are social beings and as such do not like to 'be out of step with the general mood'. MacCormick, in discussing the importance of individual moral judgements, even if they run counter to judicial decisions says:

> Autonomy in moral judgement means that each person is responsible for her/his view of what is good and bad, right and wrong and can never be overruled on that issue. This is distinct from what a public agency may be required by law to do in a given dilemma. (2008: 1819)

He goes on to say (and I think that this is important for nurses and other health care professionals):

> Certainly, people can and should reflect deeply whether their minority opinion on some matter is an aberrant eccentricity rather than a clearer insight than that of the majority, or of the judiciary, into a moral truth. (MacCormick, 2008: 181)

This is exceptionally good advice, especially in teamwork situations when nurses may find themselves out of step with a decision which is essentially medical but where it is the nursing staff who are left with the consequences in terms of day-to-day practice; the withdrawal of treatment and other decisions about care at the end of life being good cases in point. These matters are discussed more fully in later chapters. It is important to reflect on these cases not in the expectation that decisions will be overturned, although they may well be, but because these matters are difficult and making efforts to think them through sharpens the ethical reasoning and should help to lead to sound conclusions. This kind of discussion helps to develop a professional attitude to the moral aspects of care and enhances teamwork where the views of other professionals – and, of course, the patient and when appropriate, the family – must be taken into account. When it comes to the moral dimension of care, clear thinking around one's own view makes a good starting point. Also, knowing whether it is clear thinking or an 'aberrant eccentricity' is even better.

The point to stress for this discussion is that however many systems are in place and organisational and structural guidance and statutory regulation exist, when it comes down to much of the fundamental concerns in the provision of care, we are left with a need to put trust in the professionals and the wider health care workforce. So we come back to the point at the root of this debate: the operation of individual consciences. We have seen that the evidence of its workings can be said to be circular if proof rests on an underpinning and existence of a higher being. Christian teaching around conscience argues that the natural law is right because it is in line with the divine revelation of the natural order of things. It is right because it is natural and what is natural is what is revealed to be right and this also tends to coincide with divine law. We come again to the nature of the logic. To question this rather circular logic is not to fall out with religious belief, but simply to point out that for those not wanting to rest their moral arguments on a divine revelation, that it presents a problem. If divine backing, as it were, is not sought, then a different logical basis is looked to.

MacCormick is helpful here. He describes Smith's 'spectator reasoning', noting that it links to the idea of natural law, or the laws of nature, in a way which is less dependent on a belief in divine revelation, Old Testament-style. As MacCormick puts it:

> Smith effectively tells us that this is a better explanation of them [the Ten Commandments] than that they were miraculously inscribed on stone slabs during a thunderstorm on Mount Sinai. (2008: 96)

This evolutionary and psychological route that human beings take to arriving at ideas of the right thing to do can be thought of as natural law, and so is perhaps very similar to divine revelation. Ethical theories tend to be abstract; this is to an extent attractive as it moves away from the reliance on subjective individual conscience theories. The idea is to move away from an individualistic approach on the grounds that it not only lacks objectivity but also transparency. When someone says, 'I have to follow my conscience', it does not tell us much more than that. MacCormick (2008: 168) raises a similar point in connection with judgements on the right or wrong of acts. In his discussion of 'using freedom well', and focusing on how to lead a good life, he comes to the question 'How do we know what is good for another person?'. This is a very pertinent question for all health care professions.

Both Campbell and MacCormick are concerned with the question of objectivity in moral debate. Coming to the question from differing starting points, namely medicine and law, both are considering the morality of practice and they both arrive at essentially the same question: 'how do we know that conscience works?' MacCormick says that:

> there is an obvious and inevitably asked question:
>
> How do you know? How can you say what is good for me? This is just your subjective idea dressed up as objective advice. (2008: 168)

Natural Law

To conclude this chapter we return to the concept of natural law.

In biblical times Moses proclaimed a so-called 'golden rule' that we should 'do to all as you would have them do to you' (Matt. 7: 12). This idea of behaving well so as to maximise the possibility of being treated well by others is as much based on psychology as morality. At a societal level, if people generally follow this golden rule the result is an ordered and peaceful way of living. This would not depend upon the motives of those behaving well, but simply on the fact of their behaving well. Most religions have an equivalent to the 'golden rule', some value-based principle. Confucius, when asked what would constitute a just way of living, replied 'reciprocity' (Campbell, 1984: 5). This is all well and good until we come to question why natural law should prevail. What does it rest on? The answer is complex, not least because natural law, as we have seen, is linked to divine law and its revelation.

The work of Neil MacCormick,[4] writing on natural law, is drawn upon here as we conclude the chapter with a consideration of natural law and its relationship to ethics. The concept of natural law carries with it many concerns, a central one being how to settle the question 'What is the right thing to do in a legal sense?'. This notion transfers readily into the settling of moral questions in the practice of nursing. 'What is the right thing to do in this practice situation?' is the equivalent question for nursing.

MacCormick describes Smith's idea of the 'impartial spectator' as the reference that people use to normalise or even rationalise their emotional responses in mutual interaction: a point of reference outside of their individual conscience.

---

[4] I am grateful to Neil MacCormick for his quartet of books on 'Law, state and practical reason'. It is the fourth book in the quartet, *Practical Reason in Law and Morality* (2008), which drew my attention to the relevance of Adam Smith's work for the discussion of ethics for practice.

Having reviewed the limitations of the individual conscience when it comes to determining the right way to behave, we moved on to look at more objective ways of discussing right and wrong and came at various junctures upon natural and divine law. When natural law and divine law are separated out, we have a view of what natural law looks like. In this last section we take a very brief look at an example of how clearly basic law can be formulated. MacCormick suggests that there is a case to be made that 'there is a universal and intrinsically normative human nature'. In other words, he is saying that human beings are generally disposed towards the setting down and following of rules. MacCormick puts it well when he asks:

> [I]s it merely the case that most human beings in most places seem to have a capacity to issue more or less arbitrary commands to each other, or to receive them under some threat of sanctions for disobedience? (2008: 199)

MacCormick states that an example of the formulation of law that does not rely on divine revelation is that proposed by the philosopher James Dalrymple in 1693. James Dalrymple,[5] who was the first Viscount Stair, was a philosopher and lawyer and author of the first great legal text published in the English language.[6] The text includes what MacCormick describes as a 'particularly clear and vivid exemplar of Protestant natural law theory' (2008: 99). This long-standing and remarkably succinct statement conveys a generalised idea of the right way to live.

MacCormick argues that Stair's work still has relevance for practical reason. Stair's idea is that there are three principles of equity or fairness which, if followed, lay the ground for a natural law that supports a free and just society. These three principles are obedience, freedom and engagement. By this Stair means that once you have fulfilled your basic duties (obedience) you are morally free to act as you see fit (freedom). The principle of engagement refers to the idea that it is possible to limit one's own freedom by entering into agreements and promises with others. Engagements would not be the 21st-century way to express it, but we all have commitments that we have entered into – contracts, social and financial – and by so doing could be seen to have limited our freedom (MacCormick, 2008: 105).

With characteristic humour, MacCormick (2008: 105) labels these principles as 'Stair's Three Steps'. Aside from the attraction of the pun on Viscount Stair's name, these three steps have a clarity that transfers well into ethics for nursing practice. In working out the best course of action and the right thing to do, we can ask what are our obligations to the patient and what promises (or undertakings) do we make in relation to their care? This brings us back once more to the basic question of trust.

Adam Smith with his stress on sentiments and Hume with his insistence on passion rather than reason sought to counter the rationalist approach and natural law. Whilst both of these approaches have their place, there is an attraction in the clear

---

[5]It was MacCormick (2008) which led me to Stair, and I owe my knowledge of this work to Neil MacCormick's account of it.

[6]*Institutions of the Law of Scotland*, 1681, with the definitive edition in 1693.

statement of Stair. It focuses on the practice and the practitioner with those three steps of obedience, freedom and engagement. It is rather limiting to attempt to make a literal application of 'Stair's three steps' to nursing practice, but his idea of engagement, that is, entering into agreements and promises, I think resonates with the hard to define but essential parts of nursing practice which have to do with relating to the patient in a way that promotes confidence and trust.

- Individual conscience determines what is right and wrong in our own actions and those of others – how we decide what is right and wrong and how to behave in accordance with that judgement.
- Adam Smith's idea of 'impartial spectator' reasoning is a way to validate that inner conscience, inner voice, instinct.
- The concept of natural law is concerned with how to settle the question of 'What is the right thing to do in a legal sense?'. We can apply this to moral questions in health care practice.

5

Kantian Ethics – Duty-based Theory

Act only on the maxim through which you can at the same time will that it be a universal law.

Immanuel Kant, 1785

Deontological theory is a duty-based theory, so called following the Greek *deon*, meaning duty. The general idea is that good will come from doing one's duty. The focus is on the intention of doing one's duty rather than the consequences of the action. When we say someone acted with good intentions, or in good faith, we are adopting this kind of approach. In other words, duty-based theory has it that doing good is the thing that settles the question of the rightness or wrongness of an action and not the actual consequences of the action. It is the intention that is important. On one analysis this does not perhaps seem to be an ideal approach to ethics for nursing practice since we must be concerned with good outcomes and not merely good intentions. But this would be to miss the point because for Kant, doing one's duty meant doing the right thing according to reasoned principles. For Kant there were important features for a moral principle to be binding as a duty. It had to be universal, unconditional and imperative: that is, that actions should or should not be done according to these criteria. The essence of Kant's work is expressed by Campbell et al.:

> Kantian ethics focuses on rights and duties, and tends to stress the absolute and complementary nature of the two. (2005: 4)

This Kantian view of ethics is so called because it is based on the ideas of the leading German philosopher Immanuel Kant (1724–1804) (see Kant, [1785] 1953;

[1787] 1973).[1] Kant wrote in a wide variety of areas of philosophy; the interest for this chapter is in connection with his ideas on duty, the principle of 'respect for persons' and the 'categorical imperative'.

Kant's work focuses on human freedom and dignity. He held that humans should be treated as autonomous beings and that they should be respected as moral beings.

> Imagine a busy outpatients department which is understaffed on the secretarial front and so the nurses running the clinic are torn between their clinical roles and keeping the clinic's flow of patients getting to the right consulting rooms and treatment areas. As it happens there are a number of patients whose knowledge of English is limited and so some of the interactions are very time-consuming. One nurse on the desk attempted to improve matters by running a 'fast-track' queue, which by definition was attending to the needs of native and fluent English speakers. Very soon resentment grew in the room with calls of unfairness and some people saying is was discriminatory. The nurses were left with a choice between carrying on with the better system, which was improving the overall performance of the clinic, or reverting to the 'all treated alike' (Kantian approach) regular system and slowing the clinic down for the sake of quelling the unrest. The Kantian view would be to do your duty and treat all patients alike and with respect.

This is not so much an ethical issue as an organisational one. However, it is an example of how organisational factors can produce circumstances which can then give rise to ethical questions. Kant would not be of much practical use here, but his 'respect for persons' principle helps to explain how the problem in the outpatients waiting area came about.

One of the basic organising ideas in Kant's work is what he calls the 'categorical imperative': that is, a moral obligation. For Kant, if a rule is to be held up for all to follow, it had to be categorical, imperative and universal. 'Categorical' means absolute, unqualified, so there can be no exceptions, and 'imperative' means it must be done. So if, for instance, we are saying that it is wrong to lie to a patient, this has to apply for all patients and no lies must be told. This idea of the categorical imperative comes from his work on drawing up the moral code by which we should live.

Immanuel Kant's work has an appeal for ethical debate in health care and nursing practice because of the insistence in his writings upon what he calls 'respect for persons'. The idea of respect for a person's autonomy, focusing as it does on the individual, makes this a very relevant idea for those working within health care and

---

[1]'Deontology' is the wider label, with Kant being the key philosopher. Others following Kant are often described as 'Kantian philosophers' (see O'Neill, 1993).

in nursing practice. Kant argued that people have an inherent moral worth and for that reason alone are entitled to respect and to be allowed to get on with their lives as they please, within the norms and laws of society.

> The 'respect for persons' principle can lead to conflict between the duty of care that a nurse owes to a patient and following Kantian ideas of respect for persons. If a patient wishes to do something that is not advisable – too much activity too soon, for instance – a nurse will be placed in a position of having to decline to assist.

Kant started from the premise that human beings are rational beings who possess an inherent moral worth, that is to say they should be respected because they have this moral worth. Furthermore because human beings, according to Kant, understand the universe they will follow a moral code for a community where respect for one another is the norm. It is from this premise of moral worth that stems Kant's idea of treating people as ends in themselves and never as a means to an end. He refers to this as a 'supreme moral law'.

Kant sought to justify his moral approach to the question of how life should be lived without recourse to a faith to underpin his ideas. O'Neill (1993: 184) says that Kant's work on ethics is the most influential attempt to formulate moral principles which do not rest on any theological framework.

Kant is not arguing that moral obligation is a divine invention, nor that it came from the laws of society and human authorities. In his view, moral obligation or categorical imperative originates in reason. Reasoning – thinking ideas through – was the way in which the 18th-century philosophers worked. They held that reason alone can provide knowledge of the existence and nature of things. The routes to knowledge prior to the emergence of the empiricists, who worked with observations and experiences, were myths and logic. This is not so strange as it may sound in our scientific world of data. If we think about some of the ways of quantum physics, we are aware that we know about things that we cannot observe, but they come to be known through work in mathematics and logic.

Respect for Persons

In connection with ethics for nursing practice we can turn to Kant for his work on respect for autonomy. The question Kant has is: 'what ought I to do?' His view was that we know we are in the natural world, and so we have to work out our place in it. We have free will and a capacity to act autonomously. Kant was interested in fundamental principles for action. He does not refer to the 'what is good for man' question which Plato and Aristotle asked, as did the religions that followed; rather he seeks to determine how to act in ways that can be seen in the same way that natural laws are seen, which can be held to be universal. His is a move away from the individual conscience approach to determining what is right and wrong. Kant's approach to questions of morality is an approach which strives for universality and objectivity. Kant's idea of the categorical imperative comes from this line of argument. Campbell sums up the position when he says:

> [I]f any particular maxim is proposed, it can only be accepted as a genuinely moral rule if it fulfils all the conditions laid down – universally applicable, coherent with a rational system of nature, capable of being freely adopted by a community of rational beings. (1984: 75)

In Kant's ([1785] 1953) own words:

> I ought never to act except in such a way that I can also will that my maxim become a universal law

and

> One must act to treat every person as an end and never as a means only.

Kant believed that human beings were autonomous, rational beings who are capable of reasoning. Also that individuals have moral worth, which makes it necessary for us to treat others as we would have them treat us. This principle of reciprocity is by no means peculiar to Kant as this 'do as you would be done by' maxim is common to many philosophical positions. The idea is made very explicit by Kant in his elaboration of the idea of respect for persons and is expressed in terms of means and ends, as in means to an end. In an honest approach to living there are things that we learn and accept as being the right way to act; in Kant's terms this would be acting as a moral agent in a community of moral agents. In that community we know that we should not steal from people, lie to them or do them harm; these are very basic rules amid many.

More complex but equally general is the idea that the means does not justify the end. My being short of money does not make it acceptable for me to steal from you. This is explained in Kant's terms by saying that my shortage is not sufficient a reason for me to wrong you. I cannot use you as a means (a way of getting) to my ends (purpose, goals).

Kant is perhaps more closely associated with the means–end argument than is any other philosopher. The idea is that however worthy the intentions and expected outcome of an action, people must be treated as *ends in themselves* and not as *mere means to an end*.

One of the difficulties with the Kantian idea of duty and the doing of one's duty being the right thing to do and the categorical imperative is that the ideas are very theoretical.

To summarise Kant's position, it essentially holds that we should only propose that something is the right thing to do if we can say that it is the right thing to do for everyone. And when this is the case it becomes the thing that we should do: that is, to say an imperative. The point is that it is a fair way to behave if the right thing holds across all people at all times.

The attraction of a categorical imperative for health care and nursing practice is clear. We have to treat everyone who is a patient in the way that is regarded as desirable and meets the quality standards of safe and effective practice. Our definitions of nursing and medical practice include taking on the whole patient, biomedical and psychosocial. This whole-person approach to care includes having regard for their views and feelings. Kant's idea of respect for a person's autonomy and the universality which is part of his thinking links directly to the aspirations of the health care professions. The failures in the health care system, both the small and the catastrophic, have led to calls for more caring attitudes and a respect for patients' dignity from the health care professions. Nurses are the largest group of professionals in the health care system and so attract much of the criticism. Kantian ethics, in theory, should be able to provide the answer. 'In theory' is possibly part of the problem with Kant; his work is relevant but it is also very abstract and not always easy to relate in an everyday sense to practice.

That said, Kant's main moral priorities are exactly right for nursing practice and patient care – doing one's duty, respect for persons and categorical imperatives. All of these are part of the code of ethics and are expressed in similar abstract, albeit less theoretical, terms. When it comes to the everyday, there are complexities in relationships and organisational ways of doing things that get in the way of these principles, not to mention pressures of time and constrained resources. The problem facing a practice discipline such as nursing is how to translate ideals into action and to incorporate a Kantian approach to practice.

Kant's universal categorical imperative can be explained through group discussion of a clinical example in the following way. The group agrees upon a real clinical case where there had been an ethical problem which they all understand: for example, how to restrain elderly confused patients without compromising their freedom.

The discussion follows four stages:

1. Each person states what they would do – the practical solution.
2. Each person explains the ethical basis for their solution – justice, non-maleficence, etc.
3. Then ask each how it would be if they were on the receiving end of that solution – this leads to the finer detail being discussed and complications, exceptions and objections emerge.
4. Finally, ask how it would be if this is what we did in all similar situations – the nearest we get to a 'clinical law' – this sets off further thought and downsides are produced.

These four steps are a kind of streetwise (or ward-wise) exploration of a Kantian universal categorical imperative. This is the point of the fourth stage. The question is: 'Does the ethical reasoning stand up to justify making this universal, categorical and imperative?'

Moral Reasoning – Practical Reason

MacCormick, in his work on *Practical Reason in Law and Morality*, was concerned, among other things, with:

> the objectivity (or lack of it) that attends human attempts to settle good reasons for deciding what to do in the face of serious practical dilemmas. (2008: 1)

This line from MacCormick's work carries the sense of what we mean by 'practical reason' – in our case, the practical reasoning that attends clinical decision making. We have already noted that clinical decisions more often than not involve a moral dimension. 'Moral reasoning' is the term used to describe the thinking around a problem in order to work out how to act and upon what basis. Moral reasoning is used to help us to justify our actions. When people argue against something because it is not clear where permitting such an act will lead, it is sometimes described in ethical discussions as a slippery slope or wedge (as in 'thin end of') argument. The idea is that once we embark upon a particular course of action it may lead to unintended and unanticipated states of affairs, and for this reason we should refrain from acting in that way.

> If one patient asks for their visitors to be allowed to stay beyond the hours set for evening visiting, one likely response is 'No, because what if everyone wanted to do that' – we could not manage. The idea that 'everybody will want one', whatever it is, is wildly overstated; however, this is often the line that organisations adopt for their own ends. Hospital wards are in many respects no different. This approach is the opposite of 'respect for persons' and has a ring of categorical imperative about it.

A more profound example follows.

> Legalising euthanasia is a classic case often put forward in support of such arguments. For example, if we are to accept that there are occasions where killing[2] is the right thing to do, this will somehow, so the argument goes, undermine the principles that protect the right to life. These arguments rest, knowingly or otherwise, on Kantian ideas of
>
> *(Continued)*

---

[2]Pejorative language is often used to make the point, but it must be acknowledged as a factual statement.

(Continued)

'universalisability'. A rather stark illustration of how logic and emotion do not sit in the same place comes in Beauchamp and Childress' (2001) discussion of the rights and wrongs of abortion. They make the point that if abortion is deemed to be morally acceptable in one set of circumstances, it might lead to the implication that infanticide is also acceptable in a similar set of circumstances. Put bluntly, if a severely damaged foetus should be aborted, then a severely damaged baby should be killed. This conclusion is morally repellent for reasons we cannot express beyond a generalised appeal as members of the moral community to a Kantian respect for persons. We feel that it is just plain wrong.

Yet if we adopt the logic of a moral philosophical argument, ironically basing the logic in Kantian universality, we must conclude that if it is right for one it is right for all. Clearly the fine detail and questions about what constitutes similar circumstances might modify the conclusion that abortion and infanticide are moral equivalents, but the point stands that the logic of an argument does not necessarily align with our moral analysis. It gives us a pause for thought, and one to include is a Kantian notion of duty and doing one's duty for duty's sake regardless of consequences, or at least not including consequences in our reasoning.

MacCormick says that Kant was dismissive of the 'golden rule'. However, as he points out, what Kant did was to transform the 'golden rule'. As MacCormick puts it, in Kant's work there is no

supposition that there is a pre-existing moral code book or ideal code of 'natural law'. On the contrary, the issue is whether we can convert our inclination to act into a possible rule of action, that everyone could act on as a common rule. (2008: 63)

Having said that, MacCormick concludes that if a maxim does meet Kant's standard to count as a categorical imperative, then it satisfies the 'golden rule'.

MacCormick says that Kant had been hostile to the idea of bringing in the emotions to the ethical debate because Kant thought that they belonged to man's animal nature and therefore should not enter into the reasoning processes of human beings. MacCormick (2008: 63) puts this objection like this:

Emotions are contingent and variable, and belong to the animal nature of human beings. Morality concerns reason and universality, not emotion and contingency. (2008: 63)

It is emotion and reason that MacCormick brings together with his idea of the 'Smithian categorical imperative'. That is, bringing emotions and Smith's idea of the 'impartial spectator' to the more rationalist categorical imperative of Kant. MacCormick thought that it would be interesting to see what happens if one tries to re-state Smith's idea in a somewhat more Kant-like way. (2008: 63)

He explains how Kant's work was affected by the work of the Scottish philosophers of the Enlightenment, David Hume and Adam Smith. It was Smith's *Theory of Moral Sentiments* ([1790] 2009) that caused Kant to re-think his own abstract, theoretical line. MacCormick, as we saw in Chapter 4, took up Smith's idea of the 'impartial spectator', which people imagine and use the device to normalise or even rationalise their emotional responses and to judge their views against. For Kant, MacCormick explains, the merit of the 'impartial spectator' is that it brings an important corrective to what he otherwise regarded as pure sentimentalism.[3]

Kant was taken with Smith's 'impartial spectator' idea and eventually rethought his own objective approach to the extent that he came to view it as uncritical rationalism, and hence took on board some of Smith's ideas. Kant introduced the idea that human sentiments come into our thinking about the morality of our action and our reasons for action. Kant, having read Smith's work on moral sentiments, came to a view that there were two kinds of reason. First was what he called 'pure reason' (theoretical), which was concerned with knowledge and establishing truths, facts. This was the territory of mathematics and logic. Second was 'practical reason', which was about working out how to act, and was relevant for morality, law and politics. Kant's work on the second type, practical reason, is of interest to us here.

Smithian Categorical Imperative

So far we have noted the traditional Kantian approach to ethics, the approach that stresses the universality and objectivity of the categorical imperative and respect for individual's autonomy through the idea of 'respect for persons'. We move now to see how the sentiments (emotions) might come into the reasoning in which we engage when deciding how to act in the best interests of patients. We do this by examining, with the help of Neil MacCormick's work, how Adam Smith's 'impartial spectator' reasoning can be a 'corrective' to the pure sentimentalism of David Hume and so made the idea of bringing emotion into the equation an attractive one to Kant. Smith's 'impartial spectator', by virtue of the impartiality of that device, leavens his friend Hume's position, which was 'reason should be the slave of the passions'. This corrective, as MacCormick calls it (i.e. Smith's 'impartial spectator' thinking) led Kant to view Hume's ideas with more approval than he had hitherto shown.

Neil MacCormick writes in a very individual style and the aim of his work is best expressed in his own words:

---

[3]Kant was not attracted to Hume's work as he found it too sentimental. His reading of Smith warmed him to the idea of bringing human emotions into moral philosophy and practical reasoning.

> [A] conviction of mine that lies at the heart of this book is that it is urgent to achieve somehow a credible synthesis of Smithian and Kantian thought in order to solve the riddle of practical reason. (2008: 2)

MacCormick emphasises the point that we need to take account of both the rational and the emotional sides of human nature if we are to produce what he describes as a 'universal law of [human] nature'. His idea is

> to see what happens if one reconstructs a version of Kant's basic organising principle of moral thought, the 'categorical imperative', in terms that mesh with the need to give full weight to human sentiment and emotion in any judgement about how to act in human predicaments. (MacCormick, 2008: 2)

The 'Smithian categorical imperative' is the term that MacCormick coined for what, had they ever met, could have resulted from the influence of Kant's 'categorical imperative' upon Smith's theory of moral sentiments. MacCormick describes the coming together of these ideas – *impartial spectator thinking* and the *categorical imperative* – in very practical, almost formulaic terms when he says:

> We start with bare feelings, we reflect, we judge, we decide, we act. (2008: 64)

This shows how the 'Smithian categorical imperative' makes clear the linkages that exist between feelings, the judgements we make, our decisions and subsequent action. It is worth noting the differences in timeframes in which legal judgements are made compared with clinical decision making. Nonetheless, there is important reasoning to be done in both cases if good reasons for actions are to be found.

MacCormick has a rather wry turn of phrase when he names his alignment of the views of the two philosophers who never met; calling it the 'Smithian categorical imperative', he goes on to justify this on

> the grounds of its attractiveness, whether or not it is a fair portrayal of Smith's own ideas, and whether or not a Kantian purist would extend to it a moment's credence. (MacCormick, 2008: 64)

We should not allow ourselves to be side-tracked by this light tone, because the bringing together of the rational objectivity of Kant's categorical imperative and the softer empathic consideration of Smith's moral sentiment is very similar to the nuance that individual professionals in health care bring to bear when they make difficult clinical judgements.

The point to make simply here is that the 'Smithian categorical imperative' is a combination of Smith's theory of moral sentiment and his 'impartial spectator' device, which we introduced in the last chapter, and Kant's universal categorical imperative.

As we are considering Adam Smith's contribution to the ethics for nursing and health care practice it is worth noting that he was ahead of Kant in bringing some impartiality to bear on the moral ground which had previously been the province of the individual conscience and theology. When writers of texts on ethics for health care seek to move from individual conscience theory and subjectivity on to something more objective, it is common to look to Kant and his idea of the universal categorical imperative for such objectivity. Objectivity is desirable because ethical debate in relation to nursing practice has to be broadly based and not overly influenced by particular groups or lobbies. A standard approach to this objectivity is to look to the universality which is at the centre of Kant's work. Amartya Sen (in Smith, [1790] 2009: Introduction) notes that it was Smith who was 'the pioneering analyst of the need for impartiality and universality in ethics'. It is, nevertheless, Kant who is best recognised as the most influential philosopher with respect to universality through his categorical imperative.

MacCormick's idea of linking of the work of Smith ([1790] 2009: 62) and Kant is a way of bringing some of the theoretical reasoning of Kant into the more human and emotional emphasis of Smith in his work on moral sentiments. Kant was concerned, as we have seen, with establishing a supreme moral law that could be universal: if it is a good law, the reasoning goes, it has to be good for all, without exception.

The demands of Kantian philosophy are sometimes difficult to apply to practical situations. The purpose of MacCormick's idea of bringing the universal moral law-orientated reasoning in Kant's work to Smith's theory of moral sentiments (emotion) is to assist in practical reasoning when we encounter a situation which demands a moral judgement.

Take, for example, a case where clinicians are considering the best interests of a child who is on a ventilator following a head injury and brain death has been established. On almost any philosophical reckoning the interests of the child are not being served by continuing this way. But what factors beyond the purely clinical are we dealing with? Emotions come high on the list. In the discussion of such a case the parents and those close to the situation may well find the idea of ceasing ventilation too difficult to go along with. An approach to the discussion which brings with it some of the objective reasoning from Kant into the moral sentiment approach of Hume and Smith would help. Inclusion of the emotion and the sympathy which others are able to feel for those in the situation (impartial spectator) might help the more objective view to be accepted whilst retaining the important emotional element of human decision.

A revision of Adam Smith's theory of moral sentiment, as envisaged by MacCormick (2008: 63), is a revision on the basis of introducing the ideas of Kant and his moral universal laws into Smith's moral sentiments approach. MacCormick's idea was that Kant's contribution to Smith's work would be that it

properly allows for the way in which ordinary people come to moral judgements in the context of their interaction with others and their mutual relations. (MacCormick, 2008: 63)

In order to bring Kant's work into Smith's more emotional approach, MacCormick says that we need to find a way of expressing the judgements of Smith's 'impartial spectator' in a similar way to the expression of the 'categorical imperative' of Kant: in other words, to move Smith's work a little further towards objectivity without any loss of the emotional element of the judgement.

MacCormick notes that our behaviour is norm-guided: that is, we tend to follow rules and conventions and depend upon our human nature. He says:

> Our judgements should take account of our nature – following Smith, whether or not Kant would have agreed, this nature of ours is expressed to a very great extent through the 'sentiments' or emotions and passions that are aroused in human interaction. (2008: 200)

The Smithian Categorical Imperative in Action – The Case of the Conjoined Maltese Twins[4]

We can see the workings of the 'Smithian categorical imperative' in the example MacCormick[5] offers in an analysis of the case of the conjoined twins, Jodie and Mary, whose parents had to come to London when it was known that the pregnancy was complicated. The legal judgment went one way and MacCormick's re-working of the case using the 'impartial spectator' technique and his 'Smithian categorical imperative' brings him to a different judgement from the one arrived at by Lord Justice Ward.

MacCormick describes how to go about using his 'Smithian categorical imperative' approach when he examines the Maltese conjoined twins case as his example. In his words here is how MacCormick describes the use of the 'impartial spectator' reasoning:

> Enter as fully as you can into the feelings of everyone directly involved in or affected by an incident or relationship, and impartially form a maxim of judgement about what is right that all could accept if they were committed to maintaining mutual beliefs setting a common standard of approval and disapproval among themselves. (2008: 178)

We can detect Smith in this from the outset as 'feelings' are included. Also, Kant's universal idea is encompassed 'setting a common standard of approval and disapproval'.

MacCormick continues to detail what he calls a 'subsidiary imperative', which is to

---

[4]A (Children) (conjoined twins), Re [2001] Fam 147; [2000] 4 All ER 961.

[5]See MacCormick (2008), Chapter 10, for the discussion of the case of the conjoined twins Jodie and Mary (pseudonyms used in the legal case and its discussion).

[a]ct in accordance with that impartial judgement of what it is right to do in respect of the given incident or relationship. (2008: 178)

We can see that this is resonant of what goes into producing a professional code of conduct and ethics.

The case of the conjoined twins includes a full statement from the parents, who did not want to be coerced into surgery under English law with the certain death of Mary and the possible disability of Jodie. The courts ruled that the surgery should go ahead because it was Jodie's only hope of a life and Mary would die in surgery. The tragedy of this case was that left together, both twins would die.

MacCormick uses this case to illustrate the 'Smithian categorical imperative': bringing in the sentiment. On reviewing the case using the 'Smithian categorical imperative', MacCormick took the same position as the parents. The Court had favoured the surgical route: this was so because Lord Justice Ward's judgement was a legal rather than a moral judgement.

MacCormick considers the case of the Maltese conjoined twins[6] in order to illustrate how the 'Smithian categorical imperative' might work in practical reasoning. The effect of the 'Smithian categorical imperative' is to introduce sentiment into the judgement. MacCormick finds in favour of the parents, who did not want to be coerced into surgery for their daughters but they found that this was allowed under English law. Having come from Malta to the UK they were stuck in a legal system and situation not of their choosing. As devout Catholics they wanted to leave the decision in God's hands. They also had concerns about their ability to look after Jodie and her inevitably complex health care needs, should she survive.

MacCormick's reasoning led him to find in favour of the parents. The law found in favour of the hospital, which led to surgery. This was based on the facts of the case which were that it was Jodie's only hope of a life, that Mary would die in surgery, and that left conjoined both would die. Lord Justice Ward's judgement was a *legal* judgement and not one based on *moral* reasoning; it was his duty to come to a legal view. MacCormick makes the point that once a legal judgement is made the health care professionals have to follow along those lines, and so in a sense the moral aspects become inoperative. They may be inoperative, but they are still there.

MacCormick describes bringing Kant's universal categorical imperative to Smith in these terms:

[analysis] supplemented with a Smith-like engagement with the sentiments of those affected, for the sake of finding a guide to what is acceptable as a shared basis for judgement and action. (MacCormick, 2008: 177)

---

[6]The case is by way of illustration; it serves also to illustrate other legal/ethical concerns. These are further developed in Chapter 6.

Lord Justice Ward stressed that it was not a decision that could be used in other appeals as a precedent that could, in effect, say that once a doctor had decided that a patient will not survive that it is alright to kill him. The unique circumstances of these babies was that they were dependent upon each other. It is useful to note that MacCormick points out that Justice Ward at no point claims to have given a moral judgement superior to that of the parents; his is, and is required to be, a legal judgement.

MacCormick argues that Kant suggests that we should strive to act in ways that can be seen in a sense as laws of nature, laws which hold universally (in the sense that there cannot be one law for some and not others), that we should follow Smith's lead and take account of our human nature in our judgement, our feelings, and as MacCormick puts it:

> What is right for us to do and what it is good for us to do are matters that do depend on and refer back to our common human nature. (2008: 200)

The case of the Maltese twins demonstrates the value of the 'Smithian categorical imperative', especially in the emotional aspects of the case. We are, though, left with the difficulty of reconciling legal and moral grounds for decisions. The law and ethics are related, but distinct. We discuss this in the next chapter.

- Deontological theory is a duty-based theory, so called following the Greek *deon*, meaning duty. The general idea is that good will come from doing one's duty.
- 'Moral reasoning' is the term used to describe the thinking around a problem in order to work out how to act and upon what basis.
- Kant was concerned with establishing a supreme moral law that could be universal – if it is a good law, the reasoning goes, it has to be good for all, without exception.

6

Ethics and the Law

The good of the people is the chief law.

Cicero, 106–43 BC

This chapter is concerned with the relationship between law and ethics in the context of the everyday practice of nursing and is essentially about judgement. The legal and ethical aspects of health care are often discussed together. The relationship between law and ethics is of interest because ethical issues which arise in nursing invariably have legal aspects to them. The law and morality are closely linked and this makes sense in so far as they provide a framework for understanding the rights and wrongs of clinical practice and care. In a society that operates a division of labour and has public provision of services, there have to be agreed ways of behaving and of regulating these activities. This requires there to be some moral consensus within the society.

The question for ethics is: 'How do we know what is the right thing to do?', 'What do we look to in order to settle the question of what is the best course of action in terms of treatment and care?' When it comes to legal judgement the questions are much the same: 'What are my obligations to this person?', 'What is the legal position in this case?' In this chapter we see that there are similarities in the way that these legal and clinical decisions are made, because in both cases an ethical and practical solution is desired.

Aristotle's approach to determining the right thing to do in a particular situation was what he termed 'practical wisdom' (in Greek, *phronesis*). This is very similar to clinical judgement. The main connection lies in the practical nature of reasoning. Theoretical approaches and guiding principles have their place, but there has to be some adjustment to the particular circumstances of the case. Whatever the ideal moral position and conclusions of ethical debates, ultimately patients have to rely on, as Boyd (1999: 7) put it, 'the scientific and humane clinical judgement of the doctors and nurses into whose care the patient is delivered'.

Social Norms and the Law

Nursing is concerned with the care of people who are vulnerable. Not only are patients vulnerable, they are also, by and large, strangers to the nurses in whose care they find themselves. In essence we have two groups of strangers – nurses and patients – in a relationship which is in some respects unequal. The professionals are on home ground, as it were, or at least they know the rules of operation so that even in the community, where the patient is literally on home ground, the professional is in the more powerful position in so far as they are going to make things happen.

This situation is made to work through social norms and an understanding of the expectations of the roles of nurse and patient. This situation is also managed through professional regulation and codes of ethics. The latter functions at two levels: first, a professional code of ethics demonstrates to the public that nurses are trustworthy and that they follow a code professional; and second, codes of ethics and professional practice provide a broad ethical framework for nurses to work within. The important thing about this arrangement is that it is a transparent process and that the public and the professionals are aware of the ground rules in operation.

There are times too when health care professionals openly welcome law into their practice. The law has a place throughout health care; it is not always obvious but it performs a function which, in general, keeps practice safe and appropriate. Regulation of services and products (pharmaceuticals and equipment) is a major part of the role that law plays in health care. The law becomes more evidently involved when things go wrong. It becomes particularly overt when the criminal law is involved when things go badly wrong. Advances in medical science occur before the regulatory and legal frameworks are formulated. The law is generally lagging behind the social and moral consensus that emerges in society and within the professions. The treatment of infertility is a good example of a situation where medical practice and the possibilities offered by medical science have to be developed within a societal context. In complex, developed societies this means involvement of the law. Even before embarking upon a discussion of the clinical possibilities and the legal regulation of practice, it is important to note that infertility is not in a conventional sense a medical condition in need of treatment. It could be said to be simply a fact of life and that there are more pressing issues for a health service to be concerned with. Leaving that aside, it is the case that from the early years of in vitro fertilisation (IVF), with the increasingly complex possibilities for reproduction, the scientists involved were aware of the need for some legal framework within which they should operate. The phrase 'test-tube baby' now sounds very dated; indeed it is as Louise Brown, the UK's first baby conceived in vitro, was born in 1978.[1] But that 'test tube' pregnancy was the start of a long line of developments in reproductive technology, which when put together with the later advances in genetics, represents a new set of possibilities offered by medical science which have legal and ethical implications. Long before the newspaper headlines and the general media speculation about the possibilities offered by these scientific advances, or 'playing God' depending

---

[1] There have since been over 5 million such births.

on the point of view expressed, the scientists and clinicians involved in the work were asking for some form of regulation.

The rights and wrongs of clinical practice are subject to moral and legal scrutiny. It is legal opinion that settles the question of what is the right thing to do from the perspective of the law. However, whilst it is the legal decision that determines what will happen, it does not necessarily mean that it settles the moral question of what the right action ought to be, not least because there will be differences of opinion with moral arguments mounted on various counts. What 'is' as opposed to what 'ought' to be is of interest to the moral philosopher. The distinction is between *facts* (the 'is' of life) and *values* (the basis upon which to agree how things 'ought' to be, the 'oughts' of life, if you like).

Nursing and other health care professions may turn to the law for guidance as to what is the right thing to do in a clinical situation. Examples include questions concerning prolongation of treatment at the end of life and in matters of informed consent to treatment when mental capacity is absent. However, there are also times when the law, in turn, may look to the profession for consensus upon what would be considered to be best practice: for example, when accusations of negligence or malpractice are made. A law court will be the appropriate place to settle such a question, but the evidence upon which judgements are made is specialist and it is to the professions that the law must turn for this evidence. There is an emotional element in such situations which makes it impossible to adopt a straight legal or moral line of argument. The question of continuing to feed a patient when the prognosis suggests that to continue would not only be futile but possibly detrimental to the patient is one such example. The law may well be able to resolve the matter in question, yet there are emotional issues which linger and serve to complicate the judgement for patient, friends and professionals alike. The residual difficulties which exist once feeding has been discontinued are particularly acute for the nursing staff as it is nurses' responsibility to provide nutrition. It is sometimes argued that nutrition should always continue, the reasoning being that it is a basic human right. It can also be argued that if feeding can only take place by artificial means, such as via a feeding tube (percutaneous endoscopic gastrostomy, or 'PEG'), then this is as artificial as other life-support systems, and if the continuation is medically futile, then it is also morally futile and therefore unacceptable. Neither side of this argument would suggest that there should be a withholding of fluid or any oral intake that would keep a patient comfortable and meet any overt needs. The emotional response of the public should not, however, be dismissed or treated lightly. The Liverpool Care Pathway for the Dying Patient[2] (LCP) was developed to help organise the complex interventions required to provide dignified and comfortable end-of-life care. This care pathway produced a public debate, fuelled by sections of the press, when it was claimed that patients were being 'starved', 'deprived of fluids' and left to die. As if this were not sufficient misunderstanding of the LCP, it was further claimed that Health Care

---

[2]Liverpool Care Pathway for the Dying Patient was developed by the Marie Curie Palliative Care Institute and Liverpool University as a means of achieving well co-ordinated care at the end of life (www.mcpcil.org.uk).

Trusts were using this care pathway as a means of freeing up hospital beds. The emotional response to the media coverage which linked the LCP to NHS Trusts being paid incentives to encourage its use led to an independent inquiry[3] being set up because patients and their families lost trust in the service. The cash incentives were linked to the initiative intended to improve end-of-life care in terms of appropriate palliative approaches to care rather than acute service-driven attempts to prolong life – or more accurately, to delay death. Neuberger's (2013) report, whilst not differing in principle from the LCP, provides a clear basis for further debate.

Public Trust and Professional Judgement

The trust that the public has in nurses and doctors has its basis in the general belief that professionals have a sense of decency, sensitivity to others and integrity. Basic human values and ideas about what is acceptable in a civilised society form the bedrock of the society's morals and by extension those of its professionals. If professional values are called into question by the public, the basis for the trust between patients and health care professionals is undermined.

Whilst generally speaking questions of law and morality go hand in hand, when it comes to a detailed examination of individual cases things might not be so clear cut. It is possible to act within the law yet have some moral queries about a decision. Also, moral debates arise when the situation is the other way around: that is to say, an action is regarded by some as ethical yet it lies outside of the law. Much of the debate around assisted suicide and the occurrence of so-called mercy killings is evidence of this.

Neither the law nor moral arguments are precisely clear cut. Matters of law and morals cannot be decided upon by recourse to tables of normal values as if they were physiological measurements similar to those obtained for estimating levels of blood gasses and the like. A judgement is called for based on an interpretation of the facts. In many areas of health care these 'facts' will not be straightforward and several interpretations and views will exist. For example, the question of what demands can reasonably be made of a health service will yield a variety of opinions. We are used to the idea of clinical judgement and coming to a view on what best suits a patient's needs and interests.[4] In ideal circumstances the patient will be able to participate fully in this decision and so play an active role in their care and treatment. There will, however, be occasions when a patient will not be able to do this by virtue of their clinical condition or some other more enduring difficulty with capacity for decision making. The main point for this discussion is that there will be times when a judgement is called for and it is the health care professionals, in consultation with the family, who have to make this judgement. It is not a question of a simple 'yes, this is the right course of action' or 'no,

[3]The Inquiry (chaired by Baroness Neuberger) reported in July 2013.

[4]The Mental Capacity Act 2012 provides a framework to empower and protect people who may lack capacity to make some decisions for themselves.

it is not' type of response. Such judgements are sometimes taken to the courts when there is not an easy way to settle the question of the patient's best interests.

> The tragic case of Anthony Bland[5] became a legal landmark in this respect. Anthony Bland was a young man crushed in the Hillsborough football stadium disaster in 1989. He was deprived of oxygen for a length of time, which led to the destruction of his cerebral cortex. He continued to breathe without assistance and had a heartbeat. This young man was trapped in a situation where he was not dead but his 'life' could hardly be described as such. He was in a persistent vegetative state. The burden of Anthony Bland's plight fell to his family, his nurses and doctors. The decision was taken by the NHS and the family to take the case to court to seek permission to discontinue nutrition and hydration and allow Anthony Bland to die.

The case was important because it centred upon whether artificial feeding should be regarded as a medical treatment, and could therefore be withdrawn. In the High Court the hospital and the family sought a declaration that the cessation of feeding would not be unlawful. The court ruling was that the Airedale NHS Trust and the responsible physician

> may lawfully discontinue all life-sustaining treatment and medical support measures designed to keep Anthony Bland alive in his existing persistent vegetative state, including the termination of ventilation, nutrition and hydration by artificial means, and they may lawfully discontinue and thereafter need not furnish medical treatment to him except for the sole purpose of enabling Anthony Bland to end his life and die peacefully with the greatest dignity and with the least distress.

It is important to note that this case was not about any right to assistance with suicide, rather it was about not continuing with futile medical treatment which was delaying death.

Practical Wisdom – Aristotle's Idea of *Phronesis*

Judgement requires what Aristotle called 'practical wisdom', or prudence. Aristotle,[6] the 4th-century BC philosopher, spoke of *phronesis*, which translates to 'practical

---

[5] *Airedale NHS Trust* v. *Bland* [1993] 1All ER821.

[6] Aristotle's *Nicomachean Ethics*, so called as it was produced by Aristotle's son, Nicomachus, is one of the most influential works in moral philosophy. The 1976 translation used in this book is by J.A.K. Thomson.

wisdom, prudence and common sense'. He was talking about how people use common sense, or more precisely their prudence or wisdom, in order to come to a decision as to how they should behave in a particular circumstance.

Aristotle's approach to working out what is the good thing to do involves taking
account of the situation and arriving at the best answer in that particular instance.
This practical wisdom is very close to the process that we would recognise in health
care practice as clinical judgement. We may set out with a clear theoretical view of
what is the right thing to do by drawing on our own and professional values, and by
using ethical theories to assist the debate. However, the circumstances of the case may
cause us to adjust and negotiate towards a better solution given the circumstances.

Aristotle argued that the habit of doing good brought about the situation where
a person could do their best. Aristotle's approach to ethics is attractive to those
working in health care ethics because it takes account of context. Rather than simply applying ethical theories to situations or deducing appropriate action from the
major theoretical positions as to what the best course of action would be, each case
is considered in the context of the situation. In this way the ethical process and the
need for a judgement has much in common with the process of arriving at a clinical
judgement. This process of using practical wisdom to arrive at a solution in difficult cases in clinical practice is also employed in legal cases where a judgement is
required. The facts of the legal case or the clinical condition do not always speak for
themselves; a judgement is required. It is in this connection that practical wisdom
is a useful notion. MacCormick's (2008) work on practical reason and the law is
important here.[7]

As we are interested in working between the insights which moral philosophy
offers and practical clinical situations where a judgement is called for, this idea of
practical wisdom (*phronesis*) is useful. MacCormick, in the context of a discussion
of legal reasoning and processes, asks how it is undertaken: 'Can reason be practical?' He supplies the answer to his question with a clear 'yes', arguing that:

> [n]othing is more important to the leading of a successful human life than that one
> apply reason and intelligence to the course one takes through life. This applies both
> to observing the common moral and legal norms that bind us to other people and
> define our duties to and engagements with them, and also seeking to do the best
> we can within the opportunities that come our way in the domain of moral freedom.
> (2008: 209)

Case-based Knowledge

One of the things that legal and ethical debate have in common is the focus on the
case. This is, of course, true of all clinical work. Nursing has laid much emphasis on

---

[7]This work played an important part in the preparation of this chapter and the approach
taken to the production of this book.

the holistic approach to care and the importance of the individual. Medicine works according to protocols and tried and tested measures, to arrive at the evidence base for practice. Nursing too has its evidence base and, whilst there is not such a long history of the documented case-based approach to nursing care, 21st-century nursing is based on evidence and a wealth of clinical knowledge. This testing relies on the so-called research gold standard: the randomised control trial. In this way practice is overtly linked to research evidence to support its usefulness. It is, however, often the accumulated clinical case experience of what works and what does not upon which clinical judgement is based and which drives the daily practice of medicine.

The building on the experience of previous cases works in a similar way to that in which legal precedent operates. Case-based knowledge can be seen as a repository of clinical case law in much the same way as the legal system builds case law, which is drawn on as precedent for subsequent judgements. An important point here is that in law precedent involves a record not only of the judgement but also of the reasons and principles upon which the judgements were made. These precedents are such that by and large they must be followed in subsequent cases. These details need not detain us here; it is the idea of precedent and building upon previous judgement that matters.

Evidence-based practice requires not only data upon which to make a decision but also a professional judgement. Similarly in the legal system, evidence is presented and a case argued for on the basis of that evidence. However, it is through a *judgement* that justice is delivered, either through a jury or a written judgement resulting from some judicial process or review. In health care a similar approach is taken where a clinical judgement on the best way to proceed with treatment is delivered as a *diagnosis and a plan of treatment and care*. Ethics comes into both these types of judgement – clinical and legal– and it comes about through the case-by-case discussion that takes place in health care and at law.

Normative Order and Laws

Before outlining in more detail the nature of the legal system and some of its main features, we can continue a little further with the question raised here, namely, 'How to decide what is the right thing to do?'. In commenting on the regulation of IVF we noted that, generally speaking, the law follows the lead of social practices. The legal process allows development of the rules governing behaviour and, in time, enshrines in law the preferred norms of society.[8] The smooth functioning of society comes

[8]In this sense medicine often appears to be questioned by society and legal restraint is demanded, although there is a view that the law is perhaps more sympathetic to medicine's position than health care professionals might suppose. I have Sheila McLean to thank for bringing to my attention the comment of an Australian High Court Judge, Windeyer, in this connection. In a judgement on appeal in the case of *Mount Isa Mines* v. *Pusey* (1970), Windeyer wrote of the legal position vis-à-vis medical practice as 'Law, marching with medicine, but in the rear and limping a little'.

about through there being accepted ways in which people behave, ways which are taken for granted and have developed over the years by custom and habit.

Sociologists describe the resultant set of unwritten rules which people follow as 'normative order'. Essentially these conventions, arrived at by custom and practice, can only work if everyone knows that there is an implicit sense and fairness about them. We see this in daily life in a supermarket: for instance, people are content to wait in the queue so long as it is clear that they get to the checkout after the person in front of them and that the person behind is in no doubt that their turn comes after the person in front of them has been served. The overt fairness of the system is clear and everyone knows where they are. However, it only works in societies in which queuing is part of the normative order. Another example from everyday life is queuing at bus stops. Your chances of getting onto a crowded bus depend upon your understanding of the prevailing social norms with respect to boarding buses. In a society where the notion that there is intrinsic fair play attached to standing in a queue does not exist, standing patiently in line will not earn you social approval, it will be regarded as strange, and furthermore you may not even get on the bus!

In a legal and more profound sense the idea of knowing where one stands is enshrined in the 'rule of law'. That is to say, in a just society people need to know what is allowed and what not and, furthermore, they need to be able to act freely without fear of interference. In short, then, the rule of law allows freedom of action within the law. This means that we must live in ways which also allow others to enjoy freedoms and rights. Individual liberty is protected by the idea that the law is paramount in society in assuring the protection of citizens. The rule of law governs both the rules in society and its law enforcement agencies. This means that the law is there to protect citizens and, importantly, the operation of the law and its enforcement must work according to the law. This was the point of the Magna Carta that King John signed in 1215, or more accurately was made to sign by the Barons at Runneymede.

A civil society protects its citizen's freedoms and so allows them to plan their actions in the clear knowledge of what is allowed and what is not. The onus is then on citizens to respect the rights and freedoms of others. Rights and freedoms are not a one-way street.

The law – both statute and common law – is prevalent in social life. In some ways we do not notice this as it is often simply the means by which life in a complex society is governed and regulated. The law operates in much the same way as do the rules of a game or a club, made for the benefit of all and cast in such a way as not to cramp individual freedoms and choices.

Norms are essentially the rules that are followed in a particular social context. Giddens defines 'norms' as:

> [r]ules of conduct which specify appropriate behaviour in a given range of social contexts. A norm either prescribes a given type of behaviour, or forbids it. All human groups follow definite types of norm, which are always backed by sanctions of one kind or another – varying from informal disapproval to physical punishment or execution. (1997: 583)

However, social norms, role expectations and codes of ethical practice do not cover all eventualities in the practice of nursing or the work of other health care professions. It is when this social normative order is not sufficient that the law comes in to the picture.

Among the rules which are followed in a society, in other words as part of the normative order, some of the rules apply only in particular contexts. The rules of a game or a club are only relevant in the context of the game or the club. Some rules are more wide ranging and apply in society as a whole. The generally accepted idea that it is wrong to tell lies is an example of a social norm which by custom and practice is adopted by society. In certain contexts, for example in a court of law or in a legal document, to tell a lie amounts to more than breaching a social norm; it breaks a law. Much of social life proceeds on the basis of social norms and generally accepted ways of behaviour.

Not all aspects of life are regulated directly by law. There is an appeal to what is thought of as in some way a natural law. The idea of natural law is central to a discussion of ethics and the law. MacCormick (2008: 199) suggests that there is a case to be made, that 'there is a universal and intrinsically normative human nature'. He puts it well when in this connection he asks:

> [I]s it merely the case that most human beings in most places seem to have a capacity to issue more or less arbitrary commands to each other, or to receive them under some threat of sanctions for disobedience? (2008: 199)

He goes on to say that:

> [w]hat is right for us to do and what it is good for us to do are matters that do depend on and refer back to our common human nature. To that extent there is 'natural law'. (2008: 200)

MacCormick makes a very insightful point here, the message being that 'natural law' is not a rule book, rather it is the case that we human beings have a tendency to follow social norms and produce rules by which we live our lives. MacCormick's point is that it is this tendency, which is a part of our human nature, that produces in us law-like behaviour, even when there is no legal requirement for us so to do.

Nursing and the Law

Nurses as members of the profession encounter the law in a variety of ways. Some nurses will work in specialist areas where they are directly involved with these matters, others will work in more general areas of health care. Nevertheless, it is important to have an understanding of the legal aspects of the work and the role that the law plays in nursing practice.

Dimond (2011), in her excellent account of the *Legal Aspects of Nursing*, discusses the wide range of areas of the law with which nurses may come into contact. Dimond lays out the different areas of law which may be applicable to nursing practice; these range from the criminal law through civil law and professional liability, consent, confidentiality, employment law to health and safety legislation and laws relating to drugs. In addition there is legislation relating to mental health, abortion, the handling of complaints, the keeping of records and giving evidence in a court of law.

It is not the intention to go into great detail of the legal aspects of nursing and health care, as texts devoted to legal concerns are better placed to do this (e.g. Dimond, 2011; Mason and Laurie, 2011). However, this brief outline of the areas in which the law enters into nursing practice provides a useful backdrop to the main concern of this chapter, which is the relationship between ethical and legal debates.

Dimond (2011: Ch. 1), in an introduction to the legal system, notes four areas of accountability for the professional nurse: nurses are accountable to the patient, the public, the profession and the employer. These obligations are regulated through the various parts of the legal system and, in the case of accountability to the profession, the statutory regulatory body for nursing is the Nursing and Midwifery Council (NMC). The accountability to the patient is covered by the civil law, effected through the civil law courts, whereas the public accountability is the business of the criminal law courts. Employing authorities ensure that the nurses they employ are account-able for their work through the workings of contract law and employment tribunals. Here is not the place to expand on these areas, but this description of the extent of legal concerns which nurses may encounter serves to demonstrate how complex the practice of nursing can be when viewed from a legal perspective.

Dimond (2011) brings some useful order to the wide range by considering what she calls the main 'arenas of accountability'. As she puts it, accountability of the nurse 'is concerned with how far the nurse can be held in law to account for her actions' (2011: 4). Dimond notes, in passing, that there is a distinction to be made between the notion of moral responsibility and legal liability. This is a point to which we will return.

Dimond (2011: 4) neatly sums up the legal position when she says: 'Responsibility is seen as being liable to be called to account, answerable for, accountable for.' In other words, nurses can be held in law to account for their actions and no distinction is made between responsibility and accountability. These terms are often discussed as separate entities in the context of health care professionals working in multi-disciplinary teams. It is not a distinction pursued here because the main concern is to discuss the relationship between the law and ethics. In terms of legal liabil-ity, Dimond makes the important point that ignorance of the law is not a defence. Dimond is not unaware of the links and overlaps between law and ethics. She draws attention to this with the astute comment that 'each [law and ethics] is both wider and narrower than the other' (2011: 4). She illustrates her point with an example of a nurse who chooses not to help at a road accident – a situation where the nurse could be thought to be morally responsible for an action yet there was no legal requirement for her to act. Dimond comments that:

> the law at present recognises no legal duty to volunteer help and thus any legal action brought against the nurse would fail. (2011: 4)

She goes on to point out that the NMC may consider the nurse in this situation to be guilty of professional misconduct in terms of its code. Dimond's comment about law and ethics being both wider and narrower than each other expresses the contradictory nature of the situation in which it could be argued that there is a moral responsibility or obligation to help another when one is in possession of the relevant skills and knowledge, yet there is no legal obligation to get involved.

However, the situation is complicated by the possible consequences of acting as well as those consequences following doing nothing. 'Act of omission' can be regarded in the same light as 'act of commission' when it comes to a question of judgement of behaviour. Whether the behaviour is judged to be ethical or not does not simply depend on doing the right thing, but also not omitting to do the right thing. In further discussion of the example above of the nurse and the road accident, Dimond (2011: 45) raises the question: 'If she does stop and help and something goes wrong, would she be liable?' The answer here is 'yes', because having involved herself in the situation and having offered care, there is now a *duty of care* and the nurse would have to meet the standard expected of a reasonable person.

This takes us into further complexity. In the event of something going wrong as a result of the intervention, the nurse would be open to legal action in a civil action and be sued for damages. At this point the legal position is such that the employer is unlikely to take legal responsibility for this activity, referred to in insurance circles as 'Samaritan actions' (Dimond, 2011: 46). Dimond notes that in such a situation the nurse would have to rely on personal insurance.

Dimond (2011: 51) mentions the matter of 'reasonable foreseeability' and its place in defence against a charge of negligence. This is an example of precedent. Dimond by way of illustration describes the circumstances where a very sick patient is moved out of a single room on order to allow the admission of a suspected case of meningitis. As it happens, the patient who was moved died in the night. The relatives criticised the nurse for her action and implied that the patient would not have died if he had not been moved. The suspected meningitis turned out to be a non-fatal viral infection. This, of course, could not have been foreseen any more than the death could have been predicted.

The precedent that Dimond draws our attention to is the case of *Roe* v. *Ministry of Health* (1954). This is the case in which the judgement led to the concept of 'reasonable foreseeability'. In this case, Dimond recounts, an injection of a local anaesthetic resulted in paralysis. It turned out that the ampules were stored in phenol for purposes of sterilisation, and there had been some mishandling of the ampules, allowing phenol to seep into the ampule and so contaminate the drug and go on to cause the paralysis. The patient did not win the case against the hospital because it was ruled that it was not known about the phenol at the time and so the damage to the nerve could not have been foreseen.

Lord Denning's judgement was that:

[i]t is so easy to be wise after the event and to condemn as negligence that which was only a misadventure. We ought always to be on our guard against it, especially in cases against hospitals and doctors. Medical science has bestowed great benefits

on mankind, but these are attended by considerable risks. ... Doctors like the rest of us have to learn by experience; and experience often teaches in a hard way. Something goes wrong and shows a weakness, and then it is put right ... We must not look at the 1947 accident with 1954 spectacles. (Dimond, 2011: 50–1)

In other words, learning from experience, evidence and changing practice does not make past practice negligent. Denning was addressing his remarks to the medical profession, but they are equally applicable to nursing. It is interesting to note the clear no-blame tone of understanding in Denning's words. Today's climate and recent cases which have ended in court and public inquiries make this a very different world.

The close relationship between ethics and the law is not surprising; moral consensus provides the basis for agreed ways of behaving in society. The law is a means of formalising and enforcing the consensus. The moral consensus relies on shared interests and societal expectations. The presumption is that social norms will prevail and that no coercion is required. Also, it has to be remembered that not everything is covered by the law. This leads us back to moral questions and ethical debate. Mason and Laurie make this clear when they say:

It is pointless to attempt to disengage the moral from the legal dispute – when we talk about legal rules, we are inevitably drawn into a discussion of moral preferences seeking the legitimacy and sanction of law and legal institutions. (2011: 2)

They go on to say that it is for this reason we find ourselves in discussion about what the law should be rather than what it is at present. We see this in everyday matters: for example, disputes about what nurses can wear to work when questions are raised about freedom of expression of cultural and religious values. We also see it in more profound situations: for example, a recent case of two midwives seeking to opt out of caring for women post-abortion. The law only allows this for those directly involved in the abortion itself. The ethical conflict then is between rights of the patients and more generally the need of the service versus the rights of these midwives.[9]

Sources of Law

The law and its organisation and practice is clearly a vast field for study. Here the intention is to give a general picture of how it operates in order to set ethics for nursing practice in its legal context.[10] One simple way of thinking about the legal

---

[9]The midwives lost their case against their NHS employing authority and lost again at a Judicial Review and finally won their appeal with a ruling that conscientious objection extends to the whole process for termination of pregnancy.

[10]A useful text for a much fuller discussion is Hope et al. (2008).

system and the types of law is to divide the law into *statute law* and *common* (or *case*) law. Acts of Parliament provide the basis for the laws said to be on the statute book, hence 'statute' law. Alongside the laws that stem from Acts of Parliament there are laws which have developed on the basis of previous cases and court decisions. This legal precedent-driven law is known as 'case law' or 'common law'.[11]

Within the UK there are three legal systems: a shared legal system in England and Wales; the system that operates in Scotland, known as 'Scots law';[12,13] and the system of justice in Northern Ireland. There are differences between these systems but they are not detailed here as this book is concerned with broad principles rather than specific legal details.

There are other ways of dividing up the law for the purpose of understanding its workings – just as the workings of the human body can be represented differently. The main division that is useful to consider in relation to nursing practice and health care more generally is that made between criminal law and civil law. *Criminal* cases are brought by the state and their purpose is to protect society and to maintain order. The punishments can be imprisonment, fines and community service. *Civil* cases, by contrast, are brought by individuals. If the person bringing the case is successful the decision is that the defendant is found to be 'liable' (in contrast to the 'guilty' verdict in a criminal case). The defendant found liable will be required to pay compensation: these are referred to as the 'damages' sought by the claimant (i.e. the bringer of the case). These are the broad-brush differences in the legal systems in operation in the UK. In addition there are international courts to which UK-based matters may be referred. However, the intention here is to consider the relationship between law and ethics and not the different courts. Further details can be found at the websites of the Departments of Health in the UK, the NMC and RCN.

One important difference that we should note between the workings of the civil and the criminal law is the standard of proof required: that is, the level to which the case must be made and evidenced. In criminal law the requirement is that the case must convince the jury 'beyond reasonable doubt' that the defendant is guilty. In civil law, the case has to be demonstrated to the point that the 'balance of probabilities' has it that the defendant is liable. The civil law standard of proof is less onerous than that in the criminal law. It is a qualitative difference between a position where in an 'all things being equal' sense the probability is that the defendant is liable for the action or omission of which they are accused and the position, in criminal cases, where evidence indicating proof 'beyond reasonable doubt' is required. If the jury, or some of its number, have reasonable doubt the verdict cannot be guilty.

---

[11]English law has a long history of legal precedent and is sometimes described as 'common law' (see MacQueen, 1999).

[12]There is no apostrophe in Scots law.

[13]The separate and independent legal system in Scotland owes its existence to the fact that prior to the Union of Crowns in 1603 and of the Parliaments in 1707, Scotland was an independent sovereign state. The Scotland Act (1998) paved the way for the Scottish Parliament in 1999. At the time of writing, Scotland remains a part of the United Kingdom.

The law relating to nursing comes mainly from civil law. This is true of legal cases in general, although dramatic cases in the press make it appear otherwise. In the case of nurses and other health care professionals, it is important to distinguish between the legal concerns of everyday practice and the criminal activity of a few rogue individuals who find their way into clinical practice. The mass murderer Harold Shipman[14] is a case in point. Nursing also has its criminal cases which cast a shadow on the profession, but have to be set in a category outside of the everyday practice of nursing, such as the Bevery Allitt case.[15] Following these murders there was an inquiry chaired by Sir Cecil Clothier (Clothier Report, 1994). The concern of the report was with the selection of children's nurses and a ban on employing anyone with a personality disorder. Clothier's main recommendation was:

> Our principal recommendation is that the Grantham disaster should serve to heighten awareness in all those caring for children of the possibility of malevolent intention as a cause of unexplained clinical events. (Dimond, 2011: 111)

Whilst the fall-out from the Shipman murders led to changes in the regulation of the medical profession and limited the powers of the General Medical Council (GMC), it is important to remember that despite the enormous press coverage, criminal cases remain a rarity in health care. Shipman was a GP found guilty of murdering 15 of his patients and was probably responsible for the death of over 200 more. One of the elderly patients on his list, reflecting in a television news interview on the horrendous extent of his crimes and the effect on the local community, commented, wisely, that we should remember that 'he was a murderer who got among doctors', and was not really anything to do with general practice. The profession needs to take some heart from such comments, as it is all too easy to cast the whole profession in a poor light.

Likewise, after the Allitt case, the Clothier Inquiry recognised that it was not possible to prevent such a case coming about again; however, it used the report as an opportunity to highlight the dangers of employing nursing staff who had not been carefully selected and to exhort employers to be vigilant. The NMC (2004) requires students to provide assurance of good health and good character and to renew this declaration in each year of their programme. It has to be recognised, however, that these safeguards are not without difficulties when it comes to operating them.[16] More recently, after the Mid Staffordshire NHS Foundation Trust Public Inquiry,[17]

---

[14]Harold Shipman was a convicted serial killer who, before he was struck off the medical register, was a GP (www.the-shipman-inquiry.org.uk).

[15]Beverly Allitt, found guilty of murdering four children and attempting the murder of three others and causing grievous bodily harm to six children, was imprisoned for 30 years.

[16]DGM (95) 71 *The Clothier Inquiry.*

[17]As this book is being finalised the second report from the Mid Staffordshire NHS Foundation Trust Public Inquiry was published (Francis, 2013).

the focus of attention is again, amongst other things, on the recruitment process for entry to nurse education programmes and the demand that entry requirements include compassion and caring. These qualities are, of course, hugely important and necessary. However, it has to be remembered that such moral imperatives are easier to express than to organise and monitor. These traits of care and compassion are not easily legislated for. The Francis Report also calls for culture change in the organisation and management of the Trust. This is equally important as there is a tendency to focus too much on the input into the education programme and less on the organisation within which the professional is practising.

Trust and the Duty of Care: the Snail in the Bottle

It is worth stressing here that the relationship between nurse and patient is one of trust and as such it rests on a moral basis as much as a legal one. Mason and Laurie (2011: 28) argue in the case of medicine, and it holds equally true for nursing, that the legal expectations of a doctor are very similar to those demanded in codes of medical ethics. Mason and Laurie note that the basis for the workings of moral and legal consensus is essentially different. They state that:

> The intrusion of the law into the doctor–patient relationship, essential as it may be in some instances, leads to a subtle but important change in the nature of the relationship. Trust and respect are more likely to flourish in one which is governed by morality than by legal rules. (2008: 28)

The duty of care is both an ethical and a legal concept. Basically it means that we have a duty to have regard for others and to do them no harm. This is a duty of all citizens; it becomes more complex when we are speaking of the duty of health care professionals, but it is essentially the same principle. Hope et al. (2008: 51) have a neat definition, which simply says that the duty of care is 'an obligation on one party to take care to prevent harm being suffered by another'. We devote space here to explain it because the duty of care is central to the understanding of law and ethics and the relationship between the two.

The legal concept started out in the unlikely setting of a café in a small Scottish town and made it all the way to the House of Lords to become a cornerstone of the law of negligence. Before coming to the case, let us return to Dimond's (2011: 25) example of the nurse at the road accident. Dimond uses the term 'duty of care' in her example and explains why the nurse in the situation she describes would be liable for her actions if she decides to help at an accident. Where there is disagreement about what is the right thing to do, there is moral uncertainty. It could be argued that the nurse in Dimond's example of the road accident had a moral obligation to use her skills to help at an accident. There is no legal duty.

Another example could be the pro-life versus pro-choice division of opinion over abortion. The problem that arises here is the lack of alignment of the moral and the legal positions. On one view, to abort a child is considered to be morally wrong, yet according to the law of many countries abortion under specified conditions is legal. The fact that there are countries where the opposite view is taken suggests that there is no clearly correct position to take on this matter. The right thing to do is a moral and a legal concern. The abortion question demonstrates how the notions of legal and moral, whilst clearly related, are not exactly in line. Moral uncertainty persists even in the areas where the law can come down on one side of the debate, as is the case with the current position on euthanasia. Over time, the majority view in society can change, laws can be changed leading to previously morally uncertain or contested ground becoming clear, and what was formally deemed to be wrong and unlawful becomes acceptable and lawful, and possibly no longer even causes comment. In other words, the law can change following the change in the public mood, and the moral consensus moves on.

In thinking about this difficult matter of bringing together the law and the moral arguments, when we are concerned with the ethical aspects of clinical decisions the concept of 'duty of care' is helpful. So back to the café in the small Scottish town: to anticipate the story, the legal case was brought over the effects on one May Donoghue of her finding a part of a dead snail in the glass which she had been served in an ice-cream café. The manufacturer of the ginger beer, Stevenson, was taken to court. In commenting on this case, which we will come to in detail, MacCormick says that on one view the case looks

> relatively easy from a moral point of view, just in terms of relations between Stevenson as manufacturer and Donoghue as consumer. (2008: 184)

He goes on to say that it looks like a clear case, and that regarding Stevenson's obligations and duty of care that

> of course he ought to give her reasonable compensation – and then he ought to clean up his act for the future. (MacCormick, 2008: 184).

MacCormick notes that the details of the case reveal 'the materials for a confident moral judgement' and MacCormick himself regards the case as a straightforward one from the moral perspective. So he asks, 'Why then was the case so difficult and epoch-making a decision in legal terms?'

It hardly needs to be said that negligence is the main area of law which health care professionals and health care systems come into contact with when patients are dissatisfied with care, or indeed have come to harm in the course of their care. For practical and theoretical reasons, therefore, it is worth devoting space to the consideration of the notion of the 'duty of care'. The duty of care helps with the understanding of how we might find paradoxical situations where an action might be regarded as morally questionable yet is within the law. There might also be actions which can be regarded, by some, as morally acceptable whilst being outside of the law. Euthanasia and physician-assisted dying would be examples here. Whilst these examples around life and death come from the 'big debates' and as such are the stuff of moral philosophy giving rise to much theorising, they are also extremely practical questions. The idea of the 'duty of care' is a concept which illustrates this ethical legal connection, and it is a useful starting point in the consideration of many of the moral questions that involve both ethical and legal aspects. This concept provides something of a running theme which demonstrates the link between ethics and the law in our consideration of the moral aspects of nursing practice.

It is interesting to note that the story of its origins has both clinical and legal aspects. Also it is regarded as a landmark in the history of the law concerned with negligence.

Most books concerned with ethics and health care give some kind of account of the *Donoghue* v. *Stevenson* case (1932),[18] which is the basis for the legal and ethical concept known as the 'duty of care', and the case that set the important precedent in the law of negligence. This discussion of the duty of care draws on Neil MacCormick's work. MacCormick wrote on the subject of *Practical Reason in Law and Morality* (2008). This is relevant for ethical or moral philosophical debate in nursing because, far from being abstract and removed from practice, the business of thinking and reasoning about ethics is a very practical activity. MacCormick's (2008) work on morality and law is of help in addressing the everyday business of working out what is the right thing to do, and he shows how legal reasoning is a very practical matter. His point is that when we are trying to come to a judgement about the right way to proceed we cannot rely on principles and theoretical notions alone, though they will come into the matter. We have to engage in practical reasoning as we work out what is the best thing to do. Important questions flow from this, namely, 'What counts as best and how do we know this?'

MacCormick has a refreshing, plain-speaking style which conveys in equal measure the strengths and subtleties of his arguments. His account of the *Donoghue* v. *Stevenson* (1932) case is used here not only because it is a Scottish case and he is expert in Scots Law, but also because his presentation of the case is in the context of his discussion of practical reasoning in law and morality. I want to show here that there are similarities between practical reasoning in law and in clinical practice. Practical reasoning is part of clinical judgement. The processes of legal reasoning and clinical reasoning are very similar because they both involve specialist knowledge, a moral dimension and the need for a practical outcome. Decisions about what is the best thing to do in a clinical case must take into account not only the clinical aspects of a case but also the individual circumstances of the patient and the moral aspects of the decision. MacCormick's work is most helpful to us in considering the nature of clinical judgement; it illustrates practical reasoning and along the way demonstrates the link between law and ethics.

---

[18] www.scottishlawreports.org.uk/resources/dvs/mrs-donoghue-journey.html.

Donoghue v. *Stevenson*[19] – from a Snail in a Bottle to Duty of Care

The case of the snail in the bottle is to be found in many legal and ethical discussions. The details of the case can be found at various websites[20] and in many texts on health care ethics. I have added the detail based on MacCormick's rendering of the case, because his analysis of the moral and legal reasoning involved is helpful in a discussion of ethics for nursing practice.

The case reads like a cross between an Agatha Christie mystery and tales of the Glasgow ice-cream wars of the 1950s. The basic facts of the story are that Mrs Donoghue and a friend were out for an evening in Paisley and went into Mr Francis Minghella's café in Wellmeadow. It was the friend who bought the refreshments for both of them – this is an important point for the legal case that ensued. May Donoghue had a popular drink of the day, which in the West of Scotland was known as an 'ice drink'. In Mr Minghella's café this took the form of a scoop of ice cream in a glass with a bottle of ginger beer served alongside. Mr Minghella poured some of the ginger beer over the ice cream and May Donoghue drank some; in due course she poured most of the ginger beer into her glass, and it was then that the remains of a decomposing snail became visible in the glass. The ginger beer was contained in a dark glass bottle which had made it impossible to observe the contents before pouring. The bottle bore the name David Stevenson of Paisley. MacCormick relates how

> May took a nasty turn on seeing the snail, and we may be sure the café proprietor's attention was drawn to this event. Worse was to follow. She became quite sick with gastro-enteritis in the following days, and after the immediate shock and nausea on the day itself she had to consult a doctor. (MacCormick, 2008: 182)

She was admitted to hospital for emergency treatment and lost several weeks of her employment working in a shop.

Although this case, *Donoghue* v. *Stevenson*, was such an important one, the facts of the case never actually made it to the law courts. Indeed some, as MacCormick points out, would argue that the snail never was in the bottle! However, that was not the point: the importance of the case was that it established the 'duty of care'.[21] It established that the manufacturer of the bottle *could* be held responsible and accountable for the effect that his product may have on a user, however far removed from him the user, May Donoghue, turned out to be. In defending Stevenson, his lawyers chose to question the relevancy of May Donoghue's case, rather than the facts of the matter. MacCormick neatly sums it up when he describes this approach:

---

[19]*Donoghue* v. *Stevenson* [1932] AC 562, 1932 SC [HL] 31.

[20]For example, www.scottishlawreports.org.uk/resources/dvs/mrs-donoghue-journey.html.

[21]'Duty of care' is the legal term describing the fact that one person is obliged to undertake some act for another, this duty, or obligation, being enforceable by law.

Rather than go into the issue whether she could prove her injuries and what caused them, or could prove the drink in the bottle was of his manufacture, or that he had failed to take due care, or anything else, he simply challenged her on the law. At law, he claimed, someone in his position owed no duty to someone in Mrs Donoghue's. If no duty of care, no duty to breach; if no breach of duty, no liability for negligently causing harm – end of story. (2008: 186)

This, in a nutshell, is a statement of the requirements at law should someone wish to bring a case of negligence. There must be a duty owed for it to be breached, a standard of care must also be established against which care can be judged. We will return to the matter of a standard of care.

The case is also unusual in so far as it is uncommon for a case of this nature to reach the Law Lords. MacCormick sheds some light here when he notes that the Glasgow lawyer, Walter G. Leechman, consulted by May Donoghue,

was also a city councillor and a political radical, much engaged in efforts to protect poor people against exploitation by manufacturers and others. He took up her case on what appears to have been a 'speculative fee' basis. (2008: 183)

David Stevenson, the bottle manufacturer, was sued for the sum of £500 as compensation for, again on MacCormick's account, 'nervous shock and loss of earnings and for pain and suffering due to gastro enteritis' (MacCormick, 2008: 183).

In the event, May Donoghue won the right to take her case through the courts and finally to the House of Lords.[22]

It was the judgement of the appeal case in the Lords that established the legal position on the duty of care. It also left May Donoghue free to take her case to be heard, on the basis of the facts, in a lower court. For completeness of this story, we should note that the facts of the snail incident never were established as David Stevenson died before proceedings started and the matter was settled out of court. £200 was paid to May Donoghue, and whether the snail was in the bottle or even whether the bottle was filled by Stevenson was never tested in court and so these remain unproven allegations. Nevertheless, it is the judgement of Lord Atkin, one of the Law Lords before whom the case was heard, that has survived and is quoted in most ethical and legal texts when negligence and compensation (or remedy) are discussed. This extract from Lord Atkin's judgement makes his position clear:

The sole question for determination in this case is legal ... the question is whether the manufacturer of an article of drink sold by him to a distributor, in circumstances which prevent the distributor or the ultimate purchaser or consumer from discovering by inspection any defect, is under any legal duty to the ultimate purchaser or

---

[22]The House of Lords was the highest Court of Appeal at the time. In 2009 its judicial powers were abolished and the function is now carried out in the UK Supreme Court of Justice.

consumer to take reasonable care that the article is free from defect likely to cause injury to health.

Noting that the case had been heard under Scots Law, Lord Atkin stated that there was no difference on this matter between the English and Scottish legal system and continued:

> [I]n order to support an action for damages for negligence, the complainant has to show that he has been injured by the breach of a duty owed to him in the circumstances by the defendant to take reasonable care to avoid such injury.[23]

The question for the Law Lords was solely to determine whether Stevenson owed any duty to May Donoghue to take care. The problem with translating a moral obligation, not to harm another, into a legal concept is illustrated in this case. Lord Atkin notes that there have to be limits to the 'range of complaints and the extent of their remedy'. In civil law when a 'wrong' is done, a 'remedy' is sought. In practical terms this means that compensation is paid. The current so-called compensation culture, where people are very ready to appropriate blame and seek compensation, was not necessarily envisaged by Lord Atkin in 1932, but his view is certainly still relevant.

The central point of Lord Atkin's judgement illustrates the important concept of the duty of care and shows how moral and legal concepts, whilst similar in meaning, are very different when it comes to formulating them within a legal framework. Lord Atkin's judgement was that:

> The rule that you are to love your neighbour becomes in law, you must not injure your neighbour, and the lawyer's question: Who is my neighbour? receives a restricted reply. You must take reasonable care to avoid acts or omissions which you can reasonably foresee would be likely to injure your neighbour. Who then, in law, is my neighbour? The answer seems to be – persons who are so closely and directly affected by my act that I ought reasonably to have them in contemplation as being so affected when I am directing my mind to the acts or omissions which are called in question. (cited in MacCormick, 2008: 187–8)

The fame of the case lies in the discussions, interpretation and evaluation of precedents. Lord Atkin's judgement, according to MacCormick, is

> strong recognition that the legal issue runs parallel with, and ought to be considered against the background of a moral question. (2008: 187)

The moral question is 'is there a basis for a duty of care?'– why ought one to care?

Abortion, as we have noted, is an area where morality and legality collide. It is also a rare instance of the law allowing an opt-out for professionals whose conscience will

---

[23]*Donoghue* v. *Stevenson* [1932] AC 562, 1932 SC [HL] 31.

not accept the legal situation. Professional opt-out carries with it an obligation to find alternative help for patients. There are clearly many ethical issues of interest attached to this opt-out. However, the point here is that the activity being opted out of is not wrong according to the law, and so the grounds for opt-out are down to individual conscience, albeit a view held only by some members of society.

As we saw with the case of the Maltese twins,[24] Lord Justice Ward's judgement is primarily a legal and not a moral judgement. MacCormick makes the point that once a legal judgement is made, health care has to follow along those lines and so in a sense the moral aspects become inoperative, but still they are present. This further underlines the idea that moral positions and legal views are different yet clearly related entities. They may coincide and for practical purposes appear to be the same, but they do differ. Even when the legal judgement is made, it doesn't stop the moral debate. Circumstances and public opinion can change.

Moral and Legal Judgement

Everyone is entitled to their moral opinion whether or not it sits well with the legal framework and whether or not it fits with a majority moral view. However, when acting as a part of a profession it goes without saying that the nurse must act within the law. But also, with membership of the profession there comes a demand that nurses act within their code of ethics and professional conduct. There are rare occasions where personal conscience allows one to opt out; being involved in abortion is the main one.

The *Donoghue* v. *Stevenson* case was contentious in the legal sense even though, as we have noted, the moral case is clear cut. Again MacCormick's account of this brings the case to life:

> [I]n the House of Lords, a masterly leading opinion by Lord Atkin backed up by high quality speeches of Lord Macmillan and Lord Thankerton settled the law in favour of manufacturer's liability for failure to take care, against thunderous dissents from Lords Buckmaster and Tomlin. (2008: 186)

The judgement in the case of the snail (however it got into the bottle) is a useful one in nursing practice where lives are affected by the actions of those surrounding the patients. MRSA and other hospital-acquired infections are good illustrations of this point. The moral case for doing no harm is clear, but the nature of care as it is carried out in large organisations is less straightforward. Regulation of the professions and standards of care required go some way to achieving safe practice. The extent to which these professional and organisational requirements are enshrined in law was a question raised by the Mid Staffordshire Inquiry (Francis, 2013), as was the

---

[24]A (Children) (conjoined twins), Re [2001] Fam 147; [2000] 4 All ER 961.

question of making nurses, doctors and managers open to prosecution under the criminal law. The Berwick[25] review, following the Francis Report, recommended a new law for use in the rare cases where there is reckless and wilful neglect.

MacCormick points out that in an industrialised society there no longer exists the relationship between the manufacturers and consumers prior to any event occurring, such as the snail in the bottle case. He asks:

> if the decision is made to hold manufacturers liable for want of reasonable care, how will this actually work as a legal regime, for example in soft drink manufacturing? (2008:185)

He goes on:

> Is there not a risk of a spate of 'gold-digging' actions in which whoever happens to have contracted some stomach complaint can take a case against a convenient target manufacturer and either force an expensive settlement or draw them into a potentially ruinous course of litigation? (2008:185)

His point being that on the face of it, it was indeed Stevenson who caused the difficulty for Donoghue. However, MacCormick notes that:

> the moral simplicity of the Stevenson–Donoghue relationship might begin to look difficult and fraught with risk once you try to fit it into the institutional framework of law and legal proceedings for damages in civil cases. (2008:185)

These are the problems that the NHS lawyers would face with some of the Francis Report recommendations when they come to implementing them and enshrining them in law. The centre of the case is, in MacCormick's words, that:

> [t]he legal ground stated for the action was that Stevenson as manufacturer of ginger beer had owed her a duty of care as a consumer of it and was in breach of this duty. (2008:183)

MacCormick notes that his account of the case is based on the legal papers and proceedings of the case and is 'therefore possibly a one-sided version of events'. However, his version of events serves our purpose well as we are primarily concerned with the comparison between a legal and a moral argument. MacCormick's account of this classic case is very clear and graphic and is drawn upon in some detail here because it makes plain the legal and moral aspects of the case. This demonstrates the main theme of this chapter, namely, that there is an important relationship between law and ethics, and that whilst the link might be clear, the technicalities of enshrining moral principles in law render it not a straightforward matter.

---

[25]The Berwick Report (August 2013) is a broad review of the Francis Report's 290 recommendations produced by Professor Don Berwick, a world expert on patient safety.

MacCormick says that part of the difficulty with the legal case, which seems morally straightforward, lies in, as he puts it:

> the very issue of legal institutionalization of liability in cases involving allegations of negligence. The legal concept of negligence requires identifying somebody who owed a duty to someone else to take reasonable care to avoid harming them. The problem was to say when and how such a duty of care arose. (2008: 185)

As the law stood in 1932, there had been no clear judgements on these questions of negligence or how they might be resolved through compensation. MacCormick notes that the legal opinion of the time was that no such liability as that being argued in the *Donoghue* v. *Stevenson* case existed, and a consumer would have to resort to contract law in search of a remedy. This case is morally straightforward, also in a practical way the solution seems equally clear, so MacCormick asks, 'Why is the case so difficult and epoch-making a decision in legal terms?'

It is interesting to note that this case was taken up by the lawyers on the basis of May Donoghue's poverty, which according to the rules of the day meant that the appeal could be heard without it incurring her expense. The case was argued as much in the public interest as for May Donoghue's benefit. Again MacCormick notes that the lawyers were indeed:

> engaged in a speculative enterprise and their eventual victory was an epoch-making event when, against all odds, they carried the day. (2008: 186)

MacCormick goes on to note that this case is:

> generally conceded to have been the most important decision of the twentieth century dealing with the principles of liability. (2008: 186)

Standards of Care and Breach of Duty of Care

The snail in the bottle case illustrates the legal and ethical concept of duty of care. As the case illustrated, for there to be a legal case, seeking damages (compensation), there has to be a duty of care established. This leads us to the associated ideas of standards and breach of duty of care. In Chapter 1 we noted that judgements about the rights and wrongs of care can only be made if standards are set and can be said to have been breached. In the famous snail in the bottle case we can see how complex a matter this becomes when we take a closer look at the legal process. Nevertheless, the judgement from the House of Lords set a clear view of what the duty of care means. 'Duty' is a term frequently employed in discussions of professional responsibility and therefore is not alien to those less used to the language of the law. Duty of care is a useful concept in so far as it makes clear the links between ethics and the law in a very practical way. A duty of care, remember, is:

> an obligation on one party to take care to prevent harm being suffered by another. (Hope et al., 2008: 51)

This duty falls on professionals in health care and their employing authorities.

The legal system requires a standardised way of judging whether standards of care are met. The so-called Bolam[26] test is one such test of negligence. It stems from a case in 1957 in which a hospital was taken to court: *Bolam* v. *Friern Hospital Management Committee*. The judgement, which has been used as a precedent, set the standard expected of a professional to be that of:

> the ordinary skilled man [*sic*] exercising and professing to have that special skill. The point being that professionals in health care are not expected to be practising at a highly expert level, but at that exercised by ordinary members of the profession exercising the same skill.

The Bolam case concerned a medical practitioner, but the principle is relevant to nursing and indeed all health care professionals.

Bolam went some considerable way towards establishing a way of dealing, at law, with the question of whether there was negligence in any particular case. It is not entirely satisfactory and leaves open to question how exactly we define 'the standard expected'. Hope et al. (2008) point out that differing professional views exist and the law is not obliged to go with the majority view. Also, they note that there is scope for different interpretations of what counts as a 'responsible body of medical opinion'. The Bolam test is a landmark which demonstrates how the law plays a role in standards of care. The critics of Bolam argue that the medical opinion should be more open to question by the courts. The Bolitho[27] case made some modification of the Bolam position. Hope et al. summarise the effects of Bolitho, saying:

> although clinical judgements will in all probability continue to be endorsed by the courts, the case of Bolitho is important because it shows that, in principle, English courts have determined that they should play a role in reviewing medical decisions and setting a legal standard of care. (2008: 53)

Again it is the principle rather than the detail that is of interest to us here. The Bolitho case further demonstrates the link between the law and ethical debate in health care.

There remains the question of what to do in cases where the action can be said to be legal but morally questionable. Also, what to do in cases where the action is, on one view, morally sound but which falls outwith the law? Two high-profile cases demonstrate these situations. The cases of Dianne Pretty and Ms B were, on the face of it, similar; there were, however, legal distinctions which made for different outcomes. The cases appeared, in moral terms, to be similar but there were different

---

[26]*Bolam* v. *Friern Barnett Hospital Management Committee* (1957) 2 All ER 118.

[27]*Bolitho* v. *City and Hackney Health Authority* [1997] 4 All ER 771 – a case of alleged negligence in failing to intubate a child.

outcomes.[28] Two 43-year-old women wanted to end their lives, both in need of help to effect their wishes. Morally these cases are similar.

Diane Pretty suffered from motor neurone disease and requested that her husband should be able to assist her death without fear of criminal charges being brought against him. She took her case through the legal system up to the House of Lords and on to the European Court of Human Rights. Because Diane Pretty needed assistance in the event of her wanting to end her life, in the eyes of the law the question would be one of assisted suicide and a matter for the criminal law. Ms B had been ventilated following a ruptured blood vessel in her neck that left her paralysed from the neck down. She did not want to face the life in prospect and asked that the life support be withdrawn and that she should be allowed to die.

The doctors in Ms B's case argued that until Ms B had a chance to attempt rehabilitation, she could not make an informed decision about withdrawal, and despite the BMA guidelines which make it clear that Ms B was within her rights to ask for the withdrawal of the ventilator, the medical staff referred her request to law.

In one of life's coincidences, it was on the day that Diane Pretty received the European Court's verdict that she had lost her case that Ms B died in her sleep, having been granted her request for the withdrawal of the ventilator (Boyd, 2002: 211).

Singer says that while the distinction between the two cases, which was made at law,

> may accurately state the law that governs these situations, it does not rest on a defensible moral basis. (2002: 234)

Singer concedes that the legal position is technically correct, but goes on to say:

> We have arrived at the absurd situation where a paralysed woman can choose to die when she wants if her condition means that she needs some form of medical treatment to survive; whereas another paralysed woman cannot choose to die when or in the manner she wants, because there is no medical treatment keeping her alive in such a way that if it were withdrawn, she would have a humane and dignified death. (2002: 234)

Whilst there is a clear legal basis for nursing practice, there is also room for moral opinions to be expressed. The *Donoghue* v. *Stevenson* case, also that of the conjoined twins, show that the legal and moral positions do not always sit well together. In the case of the conjoined twins, the law seems clear but it leaves some moral discomfiture. In the Donoghue case, the moral case seems straightforward, yet the legal position proved difficult to draw.

Considering cases in this light shows the complexity of moral argument and also the difficulties that exist when we try to enshrine a moral principle in law. We can see that the legal difficulty with morally straightforward cases lies in the need for precision and

---

[28]For a fuller discussion see Melia (2004).

a law which can be clear, so that everyone knows where they stand. The duty of care has to exist; it must be clear who owes it and to whom. The duty cannot be open-ended, it has to be defined by standards which can then be judged to have been breached or not. If they are breached, then depending on the case – criminal or civil – the penalties will follow in the form of punishment or remedies.

No professional group is above the law. For nurses and other professional groups in the health care workforce this means that their everyday practice requires professional judgement and is subject to legal constraints. When it comes to specialist knowledge, it is not possible for the legal system to arrive at a judgement without the expert opinion of professional peers.

Nurses are accountable for their actions: this accountability is to the patient, the public, the NMC and the employing authority. This chapter shows the links between law and ethics and demonstrates that the two share a common interest in right and wrong. The difficulties arise when it comes to ensuring that this distinction carries through into practice. Judgements, clinical and legal, have much in common, not least in the focus on practical reason.

- The law and morality are closely linked; they provide a framework for understanding the rights and wrongs of clinical practice and care.
- The legal system requires a standardised way of judging whether standards of care are met.
- Aristotle's approach to determining the right thing to do in a particular situation was what he termed 'practical wisdom' (*phronesis*) – very similar to clinical judgement.

7

Utilitarianism – Greatest Happiness Theory

The ultimate end or object of human life: something that is in itself completely satisfying. Happiness fits this description.

(Aristotle, *Ethics*, 384–322 BC)

Utilitarianism is the doctrine that we should always act so as to maximize the good (whatever 'good' may be, or whatever may be good) (MacCormick, 2008: 107). Given the complexity of health care provision and in particular the practice of nursing, MacCormick's somewhat sceptical description of utilitarianism has some resonance for health care. It also, by and large, is a good definition of the theory, which is also known as the 'greatest happiness' principle.

Among the oft-used theories in medical and nursing ethics texts, utilitarianism is perhaps the best known. This consequence-based theory of Jeremy Bentham[1] (1748–1842) and John Stuart Mill (1806–73) centres on the idea of the greatest happiness, or good, for the greatest number. At its simplest, a utilitarian theory would hold that an action is right or wrong as judged by the good or bad consequences yielded (Smart and Williams, 1973: 9). The basic principle in operation here, as the name implies, is utility. Utility, as Bentham and Mill's usage of the word shows us, had a wider meaning than it does its contemporary use. So whilst the 'greatest happiness theory' may sound rather arcane to our 21st-century ears, it does convey the wider sentiment, including the idea of pleasure. The sentiment is, though, difficult to measure and this is a problem because the theory rests on a calculation of the greatest good for the greatest number.

---

[1]Bentham was a reformer and an altruistic man; he was the first, as far as we know, to give his body to anatomy for dissection. His skeleton is in on display in University College London (Mill, 1962).

The 'greatest good' as a slogan, as it might be viewed today, is fine but how to put it into practice as a policy is another matter. A contemporary analogy would be when the government of the day claims that the health service is safe in their hands (and all political parties make this claim one way or another); it is a good sentiment, but we have to ask what exactly does it mean?

Within Jeremy Bentham's original formulation of utilitarianism the central idea was that of greatest happiness. The notion of utility came with Mill's reformulation of the idea. Mill's father, James Mill, had been a friend of Jeremy Bentham – the two met when John Stuart Mill was just two years old, and Mill was influenced by them both. According to Warnock (in Mill, 1962: 9), Mill had no friends of his own age and 'mixed only with his father's utilitarian friends'. It is utilitarianism, Bentham's idea, modified by Mill, that those writing about ethics for nursing and medical practice have found appealing.

Utilitarianism is concerned with the production of the greatest good for the greatest number as the result of an action. The theory concerns the achievement of fairness, and this calculation of the greatest good is, from a utilitarian perspective, the way to do this.

> For example, if we are organising the nursing care of a number of patients over a few days in hospital, the aim would be to meet everyone's needs. The challenge would be to manage this with the staffing numbers and skill mix. The question would be – how to do this?

Utilitarian theory is popular in health care ethics. It appeals to those looking to allocate resources fairly and those interested in a just basis for health care practice. It is a theory that rather leaves out the individual. Compared with Kantian ethics, utilitarianism is certainly not universal in the sense that for something to be acceptable it has to be so for all.

> For example, supposing a community nurse who already has a full case load for the morning has to take on, at short notice, the most urgent cases of a colleague who has been taken ill overnight. A community nurse's case load has to be prioritised according to the time-sensitivity of certain calls: diabetics need insulin early in the day, those dependent on strong pain relief require supervision and so on. The nurse with the extra cases now has to re-think her morning so as to avoid any clinical risks and to cover the needs of all the patients now on her list. All the patients have rights as individuals in their own right, but as part of a collective of patients they have to take their place in the nurse's ordering of the priorities. In essence, this nurse is faced with producing the greatest good for the greatest number.

A classic utilitarian idea might simply be to count the number of patients seen as the way through this. However, if to do this meant leaving out a case that took a disproportionate amount of time, it might fit the theory but it is not a practical option. Nonetheless, the idea of utilitarianism can play out as an organising concept, even though it cannot be carried through to practice.[2]

Put simply, the utilitarian theory is the abstract laying-out of the approach to ethical reasoning that will point to the action in a given situation which will produce the greatest good for the greatest number. This approach is sometimes described as a 'consequentialist' theory: as the name suggests, the focus is upon the result of the action, the consequence, rather than the nature of the action itself, or indeed the motivation for the action.

The attraction of utilitarianism is its apparent simplicity. Another attraction of utilitarianism for health care is that it challenges the idea that it is only individuals who can make decisions about what is right and wrong according to their consciences. Utilitarian theory offers something rather more objective. Nursing ethics texts have a tendency to be preoccupied with the rights of the individual and the concept of autonomy. I am not suggesting that these are unimportant ideas, rather that there is a danger of ethical debate in nursing being colonised by individualism and respect for autonomy to the extent that these perspectives overshadow other equally legitimate ones.

The idea of producing the greatest good for the greatest number has an immediate appeal, especially for health care. It is not, however, as simple as it sounds once we begin to ask the questions hidden in this phrase. What counts as good? And how do we calculate the greatest number? Following the utilitarian doctrine, a moral act is one that produces the greatest happiness or good. If there is no good to be had in the situation, then the least possible amount of harm is the calculation.

The idea of greatest happiness or good for the greatest number is demonstrated in the rather shocking scenario, not tested in recent times, offered by Campbell (1984), through which he illustrates the point that the simple calculation of the greatest good is not everything as it leaves the individual and minorities out of the count. He describes the Roman pastime of throwing Christians to lions, this spectacle being part of the culture which included large arena gladiator sports where large crowds would turn out (rather as today we might to a circus, or indeed in past times when we turned out to witness public hangings). Lions would be released into the arena. Also sent out would be a few hapless Christians. Campbell, with of course a good deal of irony, says that the calculation here would be a large number of happy Romans in the audience, a small number of extremely happy lions and, of course, a small number of unhappy Christians. The straight utilitarian conclusion would be

---

[2]It is worth noting that there is a difference between the writings of moral philosophers, who can concentrate on the logic of a philosophical position and lay out the argument in order to demonstrate all angles, and those in clinical practice who draw on moral philosophy but are restricted in how far they take an argument in case their conclusions are seen as literal practical solutions rather than a means of resolving clinical dilemmas.

that, on balance, throwing Christians to lions is a good thing! As Campbell et al. put it, on a utilitarian analysis this activity is deemed to be justified:

> Morality demands it because it would increase the net happiness[3] in the situation and therefore be of overall benefit to our community. (2005: 7)

The ambition of meeting individual needs within a large organisation is not going to be easy to reach in practice. Take, for example, the ways in which hospital routines take precedence over patients' interests: even although for some time, decades, it has been argued that patients should not be awakened so early in the morning, that the mealtimes are not well enough spread across the 24 hours of a day, that not all the bathing and personal hygiene activity need take place under the rushed conditions of the early part of the day. A more flexible approach would suit some patients and certainly not inconvenience some others, even though it may not be their first choice. Yet early waking, the bunched timing of meals and a rush to wash remain commonplace. The overall performance of the system is arguably more efficient if these practices are maintained. The greater good is, as it were, set against the less obvious benefits for the few in the system who might prefer more flexibility in the approach to their care. The balance is similar to the tale of the Christians and lions.

Bentham's Greatest Happiness Principle

When Bentham explained his idea that there should be produced from any action the greatest happiness for the greatest number, he expressed the calculation in simple terms, focusing on the amount, the quantity, of happiness. In his words, Bentham[4] says:

> By the principle of utility is meant the principle which approves or disapproves of every action whatsoever, according to the tendency which it appears to have to augment or diminish the happiness of the party whose interest is in question: or, what is the same thing in other words, to promote or oppose that happiness. (Bentham, cited in Mill, 1962: 334)

Bentham goes on to say by utility is meant that property in any object, whereby it tends to produce benefit, advantage, pleasure, good or happiness (all this in the present case comes to the same thing) or (what comes again to the same thing) to prevent the happening of mischief, pain, evil or unhappiness to the party whose interest is considered (Mill, 1962: 334).

---

[3]Net happiness being total happiness minus the total pain.

[4]Bentham's writings are widely spread; this comes from Mill, edited by Warnock (1962).

In his explanation of utility, Bentham also makes it clear that he is talking about the interest of individuals and of the community.

When Bentham first formulated the utilitarian theory the language he used was 'greatest happiness for the greatest number'. This prompted then, and since, the question 'what do we mean by happiness' and, more importantly, 'how do we calculate it?'. Bentham's idea had been that it was possible to work out a formula with which to calculate the amount of happiness resulting from any action. He had argued that each person should count as one and it was the *amount* of happiness that counted. In his famous phrase 'Pushpin[5] is as good as poetry', he conveyed the idea that it was the *amount* and not the *kind* or *quality* of the happiness that counted. Campbell, in his discussion of this point, notes that a contemporary rendering of this idea would be 'Bingo is as good as poetry'. More seriously, Campbell's point is this: given that Bentham's calculations are based on the greatest happiness for the greatest number, he leaves aside minorities. Bentham's principle leaves aside the idea of respecting individual life and autonomy, and this is an important omission in an ethics discussion.

In this sense Campbell says that whilst Bentham's theory laid the ground for much humanitarian reform, it can also be regarded as a rather inhumane approach to people's lives.

Campbell also notes that whilst John Stuart Mill thought that Bentham's philosophy was the only possible basis for a rational analysis of morality, Mill attempted to, as Campbell puts it:

> moderate its wilder statements by introducing more subtlety into the concept of maximum happiness. (1984: 43)

All that said, Campbell says that Mill's basic definition of the greatest happiness theory sounds similar to Bentham's own definition. Campbell does, though, point out that:

> [t]his definition, however, was then modified in a number of ways which quite changed the character of the theory. (1984: 43)

One major modification that Mill made in his development of Bentham's ideas stemmed from the fact that Mill did not agree with the equivalence in Bentham's calculations, that is the pushpin and poetry point. Mill argued that there was qualitative as well as a quantitative difference in pleasures resulting from our actions. Famously Mill, in his essay on *Utilitarianism* (1863), wrote:

> It is better to be a human being dissatisfied than a pig satisfied; better to be Socrates dissatisfied than a fool satisfied. And if the fool, or the pig, are of a different opinion, it is because they only know their own side of the question. The other party to the comparison knows both sides. (Mill, 1962: 260)

---

[5]'Pushpin' was the name of a game of chance, popular in Bentham's day.

We will leave aside the question of what understanding humans do have of pigs or indeed how easily Socrates could envisage the thought processes of a 'fool'. Mill's point, graphically put, is that there are qualitative differences to be considered when it comes to the greatest happiness theory, and the crude calculation of Bentham's original statement of the theory was in need of some modification. In Mill's version of utilitarianism, we need to consider the kind of happiness and not just the quantity that is likely to be the consequence of choosing one course of action over another.

To summarise, although on the face of it the idea of judging the moral worth of an action by the amount of happiness it produces is a simple one, it is not so easy a calculation to perform in practice. Bentham's calculation leaves the individual out of the count. It was an attempt to clear up such difficulties that lay behind Mill's efforts to refine Bentham's theory.

John Stuart Mill puts stress on individual personal freedom. This is clear in his 1859 essay 'On Liberty' where he says that:

> the sole end for which mankind are warranted, individually or collectively, in inter-fering with the liberty of action of any of their number, is self-protection. That the only purpose for which power can be rightfully exercised over any member of a civi-lised community, against his will, is to prevent harm to others. His own good, either physical or moral, is not a sufficient warrant. He cannot rightfully be compelled to do or forbear because it will be better for him to do so, because it will make him happier, because, in the opinions of others, to do so would be wise, or even right. These are good reasons for remonstrating with him, or reasoning with him, or persuading him, or entreating him, but not for compelling him, or visiting him with any evil in case he do otherwise. To justify that, the conduct from which it is desired to deter him must be calculated to produce evil to some one else. (Mill, 1962: 135)

We see that Mill explains that there are good reasons for attempting to persuade a person into doing things that are in their own interests, but that ultimately, he argues, in matters that concern only ourselves we have, as of right, independence. As Mill put it, 'Over himself, over his own body and mind, the individual is sover-eign.' Mill's words have implications for mental health practices and the health service approach to the care of patients with dementia, where the care includes risk management and consequently restrictions on individual liberty.

Warnock notes that Mill's *Utilitarianism*, a short work published in 1863,

> is not only the most complete statement of Mill's moral philosophy, but has also become one of the most discussed of all texts in the subject. (cited in Mill, 1962: 21)

She goes on to say that this is perhaps not surprising as *Utilitarianism* (1863) is:

> short, absorbing and in some ways ambiguous, all ideal qualifications for celebrity in a philosophical text.[6] (Mill, 1962: 21)

---

[6] I add Warnock's wry and humorous remark in order to encourage you in reading Mill!

Warnock, in her introduction to Mill's (1962) essays, offers some explanation and response to the criticisms that are often levelled at the greatest happiness principle. Warnock says that there are two main criticisms made of utilitarianism, the greatest happiness theory. First, that the greatest happiness theory depends on consequences of action, upon knowing what our actions will lead to in terms of outcomes. That is to say, if we are to determine the rightness or wrongness of an action on the basis of its consequences (would this action bring about the greatest good?), then we need to be able to have a prior view of what the consequences of such an act will be. Often we do not know what results an action will produce. It is easy to think of examples in nursing where this is the case.

The second problem with the greatest happiness principle is that if we justify the action in utilitarian terms, that is to say we determine that this act is right, or not, because it brings the greatest happiness, the argument is circular. When asked why we should use the greatest happiness theory, to answer by saying 'Because it brings the greatest happiness' is no good, because it is using the principle to justify the same principle – so a circular argument. In other words, if when asked why the rightness of an action depends on the production of good for others the answer is that *it is useful*, then the proof of the greatest good principle doesn't work, it is a circular argument that is using the principle to justify itself: 'Why is this useful? Because it is useful.' On the other hand if, when the question 'Why is the rightness of an action contingent on the good it produces for others?' (the production of happiness) is asked and the answer is that 'It is good or right to follow the principle of greatest happiness', then, as Warnock puts it,

> one has given up on the utilitarian principle as a sole and sufficient foundation of morality. (in Mill, 1962: 22)

She argues that the logic of such a response rests on rightness or goodness of the act, and not on the utility of the act. The point being that it is the *utility* of the act upon which the greatest happiness principle rests, and not the goodness or rightness of adopting the principle.

Warnock also suggests that it helps to understand the principle of the greatest happiness if we think less in a 'black and white' sense of particular cases and actions and more in terms of types or classes of action. This, she argues, helps to overcome the problem of not being able to predict consequences. She says:

> [T]o determine the consequence of an individual act is a matter of predicting the future in a given particular case; sometimes we can do this and sometimes, certainly we cannot. But if we are concerned with *types* of act then our position is better. For the past here provides us with evidence that *in general*, if A occurs, B will follow. (in Mill, 1962: 22)

This, Warnock says, will not of course guarantee that there will be no exceptions, but the intention is, again in her words, to be general and to cover the majority of cases. It is a law-like statement[7] that can be uttered without reference to a particular time or place. (Warnock, in Mill, 1962: 22)

Consequences, of course, are not always predictable. Social context or a sociological commentary upon the circumstances in which a moral issue arises will not, of course, produce the answer to the problem of prediction, but it will go some way towards allowing a consideration of the total situation.

Let us return to more tangible examples in health care using Mill's development of Bentham's work. Mill continues Bentham's idea and still centres on the idea of producing the greatest good for the greatest number.

A simple example would be to ask how best the budget for health care could be spent. Let us take a simplistic approach to the cost of different surgical procedures which are routinely performed and paid for through the taxation system and delivered through a national health service. The actual costs are not important for the purposes of this example – we can presume that cataract removal and hernia repair will be cheaper to perform than hip replacements. We can further presume that all of these procedures will be cheaper than transplant surgery. Complex cardiac surgery will also be at the more expensive end of the spectrum, although there has been some reduction in costs for procedures which were previously undertaken as open heart surgery and can now be performed less invasively in cardiology departments – procedures such as the insertion of stents in cases of coronary artery occlusion being an example.

The utilitarian approach to this would be to ask where we can produce the most benefit for the greatest number of patients: one transplant or ten hip replacements or 100 minor surgery cases? Again the ratios are notional, the point being made is that in one choice of action there is a larger group benefiting from the budget spent. A health board might announce that we are no longer doing transplants in certain kinds of patient (on the grounds of their being too sick, too old, too whatever), so we will be able to do many more hip replacements. There are obvious problems with this idea, not least that even supposing the economics of such a calculus stand up, it leaves out the nature of the benefit and the experience of the individual person is not taken into account.

The question is, can you really trade one person's transplant for a greater number of hip replacements or an even greater number of cataract operations? Clearly not, but we should not lose sight of the fact that thinking along these lines concentrates the mind and shows how difficult ethical decisions can be. Utilitarian thinking

---

[7]Warnock makes the point that the analogy with these general statements and scientific laws is important. Bentham had claimed to make morality scientific. Mill's *System of Logic* ([1843] 1962) puts forward scientific ideas of causality.

demonstrates the need to use resources carefully, but it also points up the fact that there are some things that are difficult to quantify. The person with the new hip experiences a whole new lease of pain-free life. They become mobile and so are theoretically better placed to take responsibility for their own health. This in turn reduces their demands on the health service. The capacity to lead a healthier life, which includes exercise, is one of the benefits to the whole system, not just for the individual concerned. However, they will also be able to contribute to the community – including being informal, unpaid carers for the state health service – so the calculation is not only complex but relevant.

However, the fact that utilitarian calculation is simplistic both in terms of how it can be carried out in practice and the meaning it carries does not render it hopelessly out of place in an ethics discussion. As improvements and developments in health care and more complex and expensive treatments become available, there comes a point where choices have to be made. In 21st-century medicine and health care we are well beyond that point, and it is the case that resources in health care are 'rationed' even though the word 'ration' is not always so prominent. Although clinicians and society in general and politicians in particular resist the notion that there is rationing in health care, the fact is that rationing will always exist when demands outstrip resources.

Medical advances, which increase both survival and life expectancy, all come with a cost and some also carrying ethical questions. In the field of reproductive medicine there are increasingly complex ways of achieving births, with various combinations of donor and birth mother, and genetic contributions have consequences for the numbers of viable foetuses produced. The longer-term consequences of these developments have yet to be seen. So whilst it might not be possible to do the exact sums in balancing the greatest good for the greatest number in terms of this operation as opposed to that, utilitarianism offers a useful means of thinking through the question of where we can put our resources to best use. This same debate can be had at a more immediately practical level in terms of how we allocate our time and attention in nursing practice. The complaint that nurses do not give enough time and attention to patients because nurses are burdened with record-keeping and other paperwork has led to some consideration of how nurses should use their time. The day-to-day decision of how a nurse allocates time among a group of patients is to some degree a matter of individual choice and approach to work, within some more broadly drawn parameters which are out of the control of the practitioner. That said, there are some pressures on nurses to get through a certain amount in a given time. Nurses and care workers in the community can find that the work is being managed on a business model with so much time allocated to each visit, and gradually the time allowed for patient care is not as much as is really required to get through the care that a patient needs. This can result in corners being cut, not enough care given or attention to detail being lost. The costs in terms of stress and dissatisfaction among the care staff needs to be factored into the net amount of happiness produced.

John Stuart Mill sought to make utilitarianism more workable by restricting the idea of happiness to mean pleasure and the absence of pain. Mill also developed the simple notion of more or less happiness, which Bentham expressed in terms of quantity, by including the nature of the happiness, thus Mill added the idea of the quality of the happiness produced and not simply the quantity.

Mill's definition of utility or the 'greatest happiness principle' comes in the second chapter of *Utilitarianism*; the chapter title is straightforwardly, 'What Utilitarianism Is'. Here, in Mill's words, is what it is:

> The creed which accepts as the foundation of morals, Utility, or the Greatest Happiness Principle, holds that actions are right in proportion as they tend to pro-mote happiness, wrong as they tend to produce the reverse of happiness. By happi-ness is intended pleasure, and the absence of pain; by unhappiness, pain, and the privation of pleasure. (Mill, 1962: 257)

Mill was well aware of the questions that the greatest happiness theory gives rise to and went on to explain more about what it encompasses:

> To give a clear view of the moral standard set up by the theory, much more requires to be said; in particular, what things it includes in the ideas of pain and pleasure; and to what extent this is left an open question. But these supplementary explana-tions do not affect the theory of life on which this theory of morality is grounded – namely, that pleasure, and freedom from pain, are the only things desirable as ends; and that all desirable things (which are as numerous in the utilitarian as in any other scheme) are desirable either for the pleasure inherent in themselves, or as means to the promotion of pleasure and the prevention of pain. (Mill, 1962: 257)

I offer this full definition so that we can see the room that exists for debate around the theory. Some of the discussion about utilitarianism revolves around the idea that pleasure is not a serious moral end and that utility somehow excludes pleasure. Even when we use the term 'utilitarianism' and think in terms of 'good' rather than the more hedonistic sounding 'happiness' the calculation is difficult, if not impossible.

Campbell et al. encapsulate the difficulty when they say:

> The things we must compare include not only quantitative differences in outcome – for instance, one year's survival versus three – but also qualitative differences. Health care ethics has to consider the value of one person having an operation for glue ear versus another person having a varicose vein operation; or a short life with cancer versus a longer life in which one might feel unwell and be disabled in certain ways. (2005: 6)

Their point is that even if the outcome measures and notions of clinical effectiveness can be quantified, people's perceptions of what is of use to them will vary. And this is the crux of the matter. The difficulty with utilitarianism when it comes to practice is perhaps to do with the fact that by its very nature of seeking the best for the great-est number, some people will be left out or their needs overshadowed, or overlooked altogether. Vulnerable groups which are minorities would not come into this equa-tion: for example, neonatal intensive care could not figure in the calculation. Whole areas of practice such as IVF would not survive a utilitarian approach to resource allocation in health care, on the grounds that it is neither providing for a large number nor is it sufficiently useful in contrast with other more efficient and effective areas of health care.

Act and Rule Utilitarianism

The shortcomings of the utilitarian theory have been addressed in various modifications of the classic stance of Bentham. The distinction that some writers (such as Frankena, 1973) make between *act* and *rule* utilitarianism is one such modification. In *act*-utilitarianism, as the name suggests, the rightness or wrongness of the action focuses on the action itself and depends on the consequences of the act itself, whether these are good or bad, whereas *rule*-utilitarianism would stress that the following of a general rule is the best way to produce the most desirable outcome for the greatest number. Rule-following in this way may not always lead to the greatest good, but the idea is that on balance the following of rules will lead on most occasions to the best outcome in terms of a utilitarian calculation. (This is Warnock's (1962: 22) point about *types* of act.)

Put bluntly, the point about rules is that they are there to be followed, not broken. Even in an everyday sense this idea stands and is recognised in the 'What if we all did that' kind of response to anyone looking to exempt themselves from a rule which is generally held to be there in the service of the common good.

Beauchamp and Childress explain the difference between act- and rule-utilitarianism in this way:

> [T]he act utilitarian asks 'what good and bad consequences will result from *this action in this circumstance?*' For the act utilitarian, moral rules are useful in guiding human actions, but are also expendable if they do not promote utility in a particular context. For the rule utilitarian, by contrast, an act's conformity to a justified rule (that is, a rule justified by utility) makes the act right, and the rule is not expendable in a particular context, even if following the rule in that context does not maximise utility. (2001: 344)

Smart[8] (Smart and Williams, 1973: 9) discusses the idea of act-utilitarianism and contrasts it with rule-utilitarianism. He makes a distinction according to whether the rule is to be regarded as an 'actual' rule to be followed or a 'possible' rule, and elaborates on the latter. In doing this he takes what he describes as an interpretation of Kant's approach to universal imperatives (as we saw in Chapter 5). Smart argues that this Kantian slant is necessary if we are to make any sense of rule-utilitarianism. His modified version of Kant states:

---

[8]These are separate essays in one volume; I am drawing here on Smart's 'Outline of a System of Utilitarian Ethics', pp. 3–74.

> [A]ct only on that maxim which you as a humane and benevolent person would like to see established as a universal law. (Smart and Williams, 1973: 9)

Kant, Smart reminds us, said:

> Act only on that maxim through which you can at the same time will that it should become a universal law. (Kant, quoted in Smart and Williams, 1973: 9)

Smart acknowledges that Kant would 'resist this appeal to human feeling, but it seems necessary in order to interpret his doctrine in a plausible way' (Smart and Williams, 1973: 9).

This rather convoluted story is worth sticking with because Smart takes what I think is a very helpful approach to the idea of rule-utilitarianism, which taken at its face value is sometimes hard to accept. The nub of the argument is that for a rule-utilitarian it is acceptable to follow the rule, even in cases where it will not in that instance produce 'greatest happiness' (or indeed happiness at all); the reason given is that in general following the rule brings a better outcome.

Smart puts it well when he explains his objections to 'rule' as compared with 'act' utilitarianism. He says that his objections briefly boil down to what he calls 'rule worship'. He says:

> The rule-utilitarian presumably advocates his principle because he is ultimately concerned with human happiness: why then should he advocate abiding by a rule when he knows that it will not in the present case be most beneficial to abide by it? The reply that in most cases it is most beneficial to abide by the rule seems irrelevant. (Smart and Williams, 1973: 10)

Smart goes on to argue that it does not seem sensible to support a principle which dictates that everyone either does or does not do something, with no room for discretion or deviation. Examples of rule-following in an unhelpful way in nursing would be those given earlier in this chapter in relation to routines of care which need not always be adhered to. Again in Smart's words,

> to refuse to break a generally beneficial rule in those cases in which it is not most beneficial to obey it seems irrational and to be a case of rule worship. (Smart and Williams, 1973: 10)

Smart is advocating that one should decide whether or not to follow a rule according to the circumstances of the case; this he describes as Kantian rule-utilitarianism. It has probably struck you that this sounds very like act-utilitarianism, and you would be right! As Smart puts it,

> whatever would lead the act-utilitarian to break a rule would lead the Kantian rule-utilitarian to modify the rule. (Smart and Williams, 1973: 11)

On Smart's analysis there is no difference between the modified version of rule-utilitarianism and act-utilitarianism. Smart's conclusion is to support act-utilitarianism and not rule-utilitarianism. This is probably the line I would take too, and that said you may wonder why I embark on this discussion of rule-utilitarianism as opposed to simply giving it a wide berth. I include Smart's view because it adds to our understanding of the various approaches to utilitarianism.[9]

How Useful is Utilitarianism in Practice?

It seems to me that when it comes to utilitarianism, act-utilitarianism is the most useful version to consider; either that or we can, for practical purposes, disregard the distinction and go with the general spirit of the greatest happiness theory and follow the line offered by Warnock. She argues that it helps to consider general classes of action rather than get caught up with the particulars of a situation. There are, after all, other theories which are of more help in this latter respect.

Act-utilitarianism is not straightforward either. One difficulty with act-utilitarianism is, as we have said, that it relies upon knowing what the consequences of an action will be. In some cases where there is a lot of clinical experience and precedent, this is perhaps not so difficult. All clinical judgements rely on this and take place within the context of the uncertainty which characterises health care. But clinical situations are not always straightforward and one case may appear to be much like another, but there is variation and of course the human factor playing a part, and so relying on knowing the consequences of an action as the basis for moral judgement is not always a good idea.

Rule-utilitarianism relies on the following of rules in the expectation of this leading to stable decisions and, on the whole, good outcomes. In practice, following rules can be said to make for the smoother running of organisations and it allows fellow members of the health care team – clinical or bureaucratic support system of the hospital – to know what to expect in any situation. Rules spell stability, safety, efficiency and the like. Procedures and protocols are good examples of this. Rule-following should not be mindless and judgement is still required, practical and moral, if health care practice is going to be competent, safe and ethical.

Utilitarian principles are hard to find total fault with as they aspire to a common good, lean towards good libertarian ideals. Seeking to provide the greatest happiness for the greatest number is a fine ambition. Space does not allow a discussion of rationing of heath care resources along utilitarian lines, but it is worth noting that the ideas of quality-adjusted life years (QALYs) and the government bodies charged with determining which treatments and drugs are effective and efficient (NICE)[10] are examples of the state doing utilitarianism, as it were.[11]

---

[9]For further discussion of the philosophical problems of utilitarianism, see Lyon (1965).

[10]National Institute for Clinical Excellence (NICE).

[11]For a discussion, see Campbell et al. (2005), Chapter 12 and Campbell (2003).

- Consequence-based theory of Jeremy Bentham (1748–1842) and John Stuart Mill (1806–73) centres on the idea of the greatest happiness, or good, for the greatest number.
- *Act*-utilitarianism judges the action by focusing on the consequences of the action.
- *Rule*-utilitarianism stresses that the following of a general rule is the best way to produce the most good.

8

Rights-based Ethics

To no man will we sell, or deny, or delay, right or justice.

Magna Carta, 1215

Rights can be thought about at various levels ranging from those which require legislation to the rather more everyday presumption that we are all entitled to act as we choose. Rights are perhaps best thought of as justifiable claims, legal or moral, that individuals can make upon others or upon society. Legal rights are claims which are justified by recourse to the law, whereas moral rights are claims that are justified in terms of moral principles and rules (Beauchamp and Childress, 2001: 357). Rights usually correlate with duties. They can also conflict with the rights of others. For example, a patient may ask to exercise their right to discharge themself from hospital too soon after major surgery, an action clearly against their clinical interests. It might be within a patient's rights to ask to do this, but a duty of care is likely to prevent the nurse or doctor from going along with the idea.

Rights-based ethical theory is attractive as it serves the individual's rights, but it has to be remembered that these are not absolute. There is a balance to be struck with the rights of others; this balance is a useful corrective to the impression, sometimes given in nursing ethics texts, that individualism is paramount. Nursing ethics has been to an extent colonised by autonomy as an organising principle. If individual autonomy is the driving principle, it sets up a rather unrealistic situation in which ethics for nursing practice is discussed in a moral vacuum, with too much emphasis on the individual and insufficient regard for the immediate community or the wider society. Mason and Laurie (2011: 7) make a similar point and note that communitarianism[1] is gaining ground as something of 'a counterweight to the almost relentlessly

---

[1]Communitarianism is an ethical theory focusing on social justice and less on individual rights. In practical terms, it judges the action by the good or bad effect on the society, not the individual per se.

increasing reliance on personal autonomy as a cornerstone to both medical ethics and medical law'.

Rights can be positive, such as when someone is provided with a service. Or rights can be negative: that is to say, a person can demand that someone desists from doing them harm or causing them inconvenience. In our daily lives we make the assumption that so long as our behaviour comes within the limits of the law we can act as we choose. There are, of course, constraints placed upon us by social and family commitments and the demands of work, but these aside we are free to act as we please. The presumption is that we are all autonomous beings and, in Kant's terms, we deserve to be respected as autonomous moral beings. The rule of law allows freedom of action within the law and, importantly, ensures that individuals are aware of what they can and cannot do within the law. This means that we must live in ways which also allow others to enjoy freedoms and rights, but that within these constraints we are autonomous.

It is commonplace to discuss health care in the language of rights. People speak of there being rights to care, to treatment, to privacy, choice and so on. On closer examination we can see that rights are not uncomplicated and neither are they absolute. The libertarian instincts of a developed country tend to produce an approach to health care which is similar to the approach taken to the provision of other goods and services. In health care there is an increasing tendency to approach the matter as one might any other service industry which includes a concern for choice and quality and some recompense if all is not as it should be when the service is delivered. A business model works on the basis of there being a contract between the service provider and the customer, there are rights and expectations built into this model and a system for remedy and compensation when things do not go to plan. Rights-based ethical theory when applied to individual clinical cases takes us into moral territory and points up the difficulties of using a business contractual approach to health care, which is, of course, a deal more complex.

Rights and Treatment in an Institution

Patients have a right to competent safe treatment. A competent adult patient can refuse any treatment as of right. Where there is a question of lack of mental capacity, the Mental Capacity Act (2005)[2] sets out how a person's best interests can be determined, and applies to people aged 16 and over. The general principle enshrined in the Act is that there must be equal consideration, which means that no factor such as age, appearance or disability can be used as a reason why the person cannot make a decision. McLean says:

> It is generally agreed that the corollary of the right to consent to treatment is the right to refuse it. While choosing to accept recommended therapy can be an affirmation of

---

[2]Consent and capacity is a complex matter. For details, see Dimond (2011) and Mason and Laurie (2011).

the patient's autonomy, so too can his/her decision to avoid or reject it. Both are about self-determination or control over our lives. (2010: 99)

We have noted that within the constraints of the law and the demands made of us, because we co-exist with others in society we are free to choose how we go about our business. This freedom is not available to everyone. Leaving aside those in prison, there are those who are not at liberty to run their own lives. Those who rely on others for their care, physical and social, cannot be said to be as free as those able to not only plan but also carry out their plans unaided. If we are dependent upon others for our daily needs, it is a consequence of that situation that we are dependent upon others for our freedom of action in daily life. People with a physical disability have to rely on carers in order to function. The more severe the disability, the higher the dependency. When a patient is in hospital there are restrictions on freedom. This is, to an extent, a consequence of institutional life.

> A man in his late eighties recovering from bronchitis, the latest episode of many, tells the nurses that he does not feel like eating and is happy to be left to rest. The charge nurse thinks that he should just be given drinks and asks the nursing staff not to press him to eat if he continues to show no interest in food. However, the following day the staff nurse takes over charge of the ward and says that all he needs is encouragement to resume eating and asks a student nurse to help him with lunch. He is very distressed by this intervention as he is not in need of physical help, and the student feels very strongly that she should not have been asked to offer food against his express wish to the contrary. The staff nurse justifies her decision by saying that nurses have a duty of care and this includes ensuring that patients are nourished.

This case causes us to stop and ask at least two questions. Are there occasions when nurses should put patients' wishes before their well-being? Are nurses justified in making decisions for patients just because they have been admitted to hospital?

In this case it is the principles of beneficence and non-maleficence that might be driving the staff nurse's decision. The duty of care also plays a part. But these considerations have to be set against the good that might come from adhering to the man's wishes. Rights-based ethics would put this as a priority. He may simply have had enough and has come to the view that he just wants nature to take its course.[3] This case only moves into the moral arena because the man is in hospital. If he were in his own home, he would be free of the professionals' duty of care and of the Hospital Trust's vicarious responsibility for his welfare. Put in simple terms, he would be free to do as he wished, and need give no thought to the views of others on the matter.

---

[3]For further discussion of options of last resort, see Melia (2011). About decision making at the end of life, see the case commentary in *Asian Bioethics Review*, June 2011, 3(2): 145–9.

This fact points up just how restricted some rights can be. If you were to ask yourself 'How do I justify feeding or not feeding this man, who does not want to eat?', you would, in a very practical sense, be right in the midst of a debate about beneficence versus non-maleficence and, for good measure, principles of justice and rights would also be to the fore.

In institutions such as hospitals or care homes, rules of the organisation take priority when it comes to risk avoidance. This will have an effect on freedom of decisions and actions. How far should a hospital go with its measures to maintain patient safety? The unintended consequences of over-caution could result in patients' rights being infringed, leading to frustration and distress. If there are in fact few accidents occurring when patients are free to move around unhindered by safety measures, then it would be reasonable to allow the freedom and benefit from the improvement in mood and quality of daily life that ensues. If, on the other hand, the freedom to move around is the greater hazard, then preventive measures make sense and will produce a better environment with less injury, even if it is at the cost of limiting freedom. It is in this very everyday sense that rights can be gradually eroded.

Unfortunately, there is a tendency for institutions to resort to general rules and bureaucratic solutions to individual situations, and this leads to a situation in which the autonomy of some patients will seem to be respected more readily than is the case with others. A younger, fitter person who is aware of their surroundings would doubtless be accorded more freedom. On the face of it, this commonplace matter might be regarded as unimportant. Yet, basic questions of freedom to choose and to act are ultimately questions of rights. During a short stay in hospital the lack of freedom and autonomy may not give rise to much concern, although we might ask why not. Is there a moral difference between short- and long-term stay, or is it simply more socially acceptable? If we consider the long-stay cases or the permanent care home situation, then whilst the basic right does not alter, the compromise of these underlying ethical principles does give cause for concern.

A rights-based ethical theory is essentially about outlining the rules that can be enforced by society and which should be followed by members of that society. It is not a list of entitlements, rather a starting point for mutual co-operation in a democratic society. The rights-based approach to ethics fits well with the 21st-century approach to health care. The modernised NHS puts the patient in the centre and seeks to organise the service around the needs and lifestyles of patients, rather than allowing professional needs to determine the ways in which the service is organised.

There are the rights of the health care workers to be considered, but how far do these extend?

Take, for example, the case of the two Catholic midwives who sought leave to refuse to supervise or support staff who were involved in the care of women undergoing abortions. They claimed that being required to supervise staff involved in abortion was a violation of their human rights. The Abortion Act (1967) provides for one of the few areas in health care where professionals are able to opt out of direct care on moral grounds, provided that they ensure that alternative care is provided for the patient. Their case failed because the judgement was that the right to opt out on moral grounds only applies to the 'frontline' of the service. The hospital accepts that midwives may opt out of hands-on involvement in the procedures, but holds that midwifery sisters cannot opt out of their role of 'delegation, supervision and support' of midwives carrying out the abortion procedures. The fact that these midwives were not involved in the abortion procedure itself, and therefore not in the frontline, meant that they did not have grounds to opt out of the care.

The case demonstrates the balance that is needed between the professional's freedom of conscience with the woman's right to terminate a pregnancy through the legally sanctioned procedures. The individual rights of the professionals are set against the need to have a system that works for all. The Judge's view was that as there is no compulsion to be a midwife and so long as the involvement is not directly with the abortion, then they have to 'get on with the job'.

Industrial action is an example of the juxtaposition of one group's rights and those of another.

There are several features of rights which make them less straightforward than they might at first appear to be. Rights are discussed at various levels of formality. In everyday speech we might say, 'I have a right to x because I have done y'.

A member of the nursing staff may have worked over a holiday weekend in order to allow colleagues with children to take the public holiday off in order to be with the family. The nurse who has worked the shift may imply or state overtly that she has a right to take the next weekend off in return. Even if it is not stated, the implication is that she has a moral right to the days off in return for her earlier sacrifice of the holiday weekend.

In ethical debate, moral theories are drawn upon rather than the tit-for-tat approach adopted in this example.

Ethical principles which can be appealed to in justifying a right can be in conflict. It is interesting to note that the same principle is sometimes called upon for the justification of both sides of an ethical debate. For example, respect for a person's dignity and autonomy is usually given as the ethical reasoning behind the call for the right of a person to end their own life at a time of their choosing – assisted dying. Paradoxically, it is respect for human dignity that is called upon in support of the opposite view. The same can be seen in the pro-life and pro-choice debate around abortion: dignity is called upon to support rights of the mother and of the child.

Uncertainty and Rights

Uncertainty and unpredictability characterise heath care. We should always be ready for the unexpected prognosis but equally aware that expectations are not always played out. 'You have six months to live' is a line much more likely to be delivered from the theatre stage than in any medical consulting room. Medical prognoses are discussed in terms of what might be expected with reference to typical cases and a clinician's experience in order to give people a chance to plan to use the remaining time in the light of their diagnosis. For patients living longer than was expected there can be various consequences. It can be a bonus, or it can lead to ethical questions when it is not a welcome extension and a desire to end life is seriously contemplated. Alongside this uncertainty we have increasing numbers of people calling for the right to choose when their life should end.

During the analysis of interview data in a study of the ethical issues in intensive care (see Melia, 2004: Ch. 3), the relationship between care, cure and palliation was explored and characterised as the care–cure–palliation triangle with each side having a connection to the other, whilst at the same time being seen as separate entities. The sides of the triangle are related and a movement in one direction has consequences in another. For example, a decision to give 'nursing care only' may overlook the cure potential. One question that this kind of analysis raises is, 'Can burdensome treatments can be justified on palliative grounds?' If the intention was to effect a cure or a remission and it failed, was the patient in some ways in a worse position than if such an approach had not been adopted in the first place? Might a palliative approach been a better option in the long run? Hovering over this discussion is the ever-present problem of uncertainty.

Space does not allow further discussion here, save to note that this kind of thinking is helpful in relation to the Liverpool Care Pathway, which has given rise to misunderstandings about the intentions and has resulted in the unintended consequence of denting public trust in the health service in this sensitive area (see Chapter 3).

Euthanasia and Assisted Dying

Uncertainty has also entered the terminology around euthanasia and assisted dying. The discussion of the end of life has moved up the public agenda, and indeed there is active encouragement of people to openly discuss their views on and wishes for end-of-life care. The reasons for this are various, mostly to make end-of-life care more appropriate,[4] but also to facilitate more organ donation to supply the transplant service where there are more people waiting for organs than there are donors.

The language around end-of-life has become confused. The original meaning of 'euthanasia' (from the Greek *thanatos*, meaning 'death') was literally a good or easy

---

[4]Delivering Dignity (2012).

death and goes back to the time of Hippocrates, who thought that a good death was what medicine should strive for when a cure is not possible. More recently euthanasia has come to mean ending life. It is illegal for doctors, nurses (anyone, in fact) to assist in ending a life. Even helping someone travel to Switzerland to use the services of Dignitas[5] brings a person, professional or friend, into the situation where they might be questioned by the police. The Swiss are reported to be unhappy with the way in which countries where assisted dying is illegal are using Switzerland for what might be termed an 'offshore' end-of-life service.

Uncertainty has also crept into the terminology in discussions about the right to determine when to end life when more than cessation of treatment is required. The term 'euthanasia', Mason and Laurie say, is being used in a broader sense than the narrower concept should allow. Mason and Laurie say that they want as far as possible:

> to eliminate the use of the word 'euthanasia' from any variation on 'assisted dying' that does not involve intentional shorting of life – or what is becoming known as 'therapeutic killing' (2011: 565)[6]

We have to remember that the social context is as important as the factual base. For example, when in 2009 the Royal College of Nursing, following a members' vote, dropped its five-year opposition to the principle of assisted suicide, the College position changed to 'a neutral stance'. Whilst this position is clearly different from supporting assisted suicide, the nature of news reporting makes the statement vulnerable to misinterpretation. At the same time the British Medical Association stood by their opposition to assisted suicide (see British Medical Association, 2009: Ch. 11). This is perhaps not surprising as doctors are the most likely among the health care professions to be asked to assist a patient who wants to die.

We could mount an argument that says health professionals should have nothing to do with euthanasia in any guise. The argument would go like this: it may be that it is in the interests of a patient that his life is ended, but there is no reason why medicine and nursing should become involved. However, this argument is not likely to carry much weight, especially in the context of a society which is beginning to reappraise the end of life and how its institutions propose to handle the changes in attitude towards end of life and end-of-life options. There is a comparison to be made between euthanasia and abortion. In the early days of abortion law reform, the medical profession became involved at least in part because the alternative back-street practice did more harm than would a properly run abortion service. A similar situation could arise with euthanasia. Indeed, some might argue that it already has, with the various organisations and internet sites that give information on how to

---

[5]The Swiss-based clinic which provides assisted dying. This is legal in Switzerland.

[6]For further discussion of this point, see Mason and Laurie (2011), Chapter 18.

end life.[7] It seems then to be the case that, like it or not, health care professionals are obliged at least to consider their position on euthanasia.

Even with the general changing of attitudes towards how we approach the end of life, the question of whether there is a right to die comes under the eye of the law.[8] As we have seen, there are situations where the moral case for an action is made, but the legal position does not always follow the same line of reasoning or arrive at the same conclusion. When no more clinical options exist and a patient is dying, there is no legal requirement for treatment to continue because to prolong a life is not in the patient's interests. Or even if it is deemed to be in the patients' interests by the clinicians but the patient does not wish to continue, there is no requirement to carry on with treatment. Indeed, if the patient is fully capable of deciding what they want to happen, they can refuse any treatment at any time.

Rights Consent and Confidentiality

Among the rights patients have is the right to confidentiality. There are exceptions to this general rule of confidentiality to which professionals must adhere. These are when the patient gives permission to break confidence, or when it is in the patient's interests: for example, when disclosing to another professional in the best interests of the patient's care. Or it may be in the public interest, when the grounds rest on questions of public safety. The public interest is an interesting question as little has been tested in the courts.[9]

The principle of consent is the means by which patients' rights are safeguarded. Both the law of consent and the ethical principle of consent are underpinned by one of the four principles (see Chapter 2), namely, respect for autonomy. Informed consent, or informed choice (a less paternalistic term), is one of the main ways in which the principle of respect for autonomy works in practice. Patients are entitled to have control over their lives and so with any proposed medical intervention there has to be patient consent. It is a consent described as informed, meaning that the patient

---

[7]Using the expression 'commit suicide' seems to be less acceptable in the 21st century, not least because since suicide is no longer a criminal act, the verb 'to commit' is not appropriate. 'Assisted dying' is becoming the term that is replacing physician-assisted suicide and euthanasia.

[8]In England and Wales the Commission on Assisted Dying was set up in 2010 to consider whether the legal and policy approaches to assisted dying are appropriate, and working and to evaluate the legal status quo. The Commission's main conclusion was that 'the current legal status of assisted suicide is inadequate and incoherent' (Report of the Commission on Assisted Dying, Demos, 2011, www.demos.co.uk).

[9]See Dimond (2011), Chapter 8, for discussion of the legal position. The inclusion in this discussion of rights-based ethics is to demonstrate that rights are not always as clear cut as we might suppose. See also Hope et al. (2008).

has been made aware of the implications of the treatment, positive and negative, and of the risk involved. In other words, their consent if given must be an informed choice. It should go without saying that consent must be voluntary.

When it comes to consent to treatment, once a patient has decided that they do not want treatment or the continuation of treatment (assuming their mental capacity is such that they can make a decision), then that decision is binding on the medical staff. Doctors are obliged, by the medical professional code and by law, to accept the decision and not treat.[10]

McLean says that we may be troubled by decisions others make not to continue with life when it would have been possible to continue. We have to accept that when people have autonomy, this is what it can mean. Sometimes health care professionals have to arrive at an idea of what we think the patient's best interests would be. This is not always in situations of life or death, but in the circumstances when a patient is unconscious or otherwise unable to express themselves and we take care of the needs that they would normally attend to themselves – in small and greater ways we make decisions on their behalf. A patient recovering from a stroke is very dependent upon nursing staff as they gradually gain their confidence to face the world. Nurses taking time and consideration to ensure that they look as good as they can are, in effect, supporting autonomy which has been partially restored and has to be fully regained.

In the context of having to accept that the autonomy of a patient may lead to uncomfortable situations, McLean makes the following point that well sums up the position in which nurses can find themselves:

> While it is almost certainly the case that most people value every second of their lives, there are some for whom life has become intolerable and/or unwanted. We may not understand why this is so, nor may we believe that in their circumstances we would feel the same way, but the value attributed to one's own life is a highly personal matter which is not susceptible of second-guessing by others. Having said that, the state, through the vehicle of the law, claims an interest in preserving life; an interest that, in most countries throughout the world, means that the law prohibits assisted dying (either assisted suicide or voluntary euthanasia). Killing is universally regarded as wrong. (2010: 99)

In this statement McLean covers the main points, both legal and ethical, in this complex area. It is worth noting at this juncture that the law does not regard withdrawal of treatment as a category of 'killing', that is to say it is not regarded as active euthanasia. In other words, withholding treatment and withdrawing treatment are legally speaking in the same category (Hope et al., 2008: 180).

Difficulties arise when patients are unable to state their wishes either due to their clinical state or because of a lack of mental capacity. The question of whether life should go on does not always come at the end of a long life: the situation can arise in the much more dramatic circumstances of very major trauma and what can properly be described as horrendous injury. This takes us into the realms of ethical dilemma, which as we have

---

[10]For a fuller discussion, see Mason and Laurie (2011).

noted can help to sharpen the issues in the debate and so be useful in thinking through the more everyday moral choice situations that are much more generally to be found.

This next example is extreme, but the principle is more broadly applicable given the advanced state of medical technology and the possibilities thus opened up.

> There is, according to the US Army medical services, a new category of patient coming back to hospitals in the United States from the war zones, notably Afghanistan. The category is 'the unexpected survivor'. As we have noted, the uncertainty that exists around prognosis, and those who, in the words of the popular press, 'cheat death', might be thought of as 'unexpected survivors'. However, the meaning of this 'unexpected survivor' label given to the soldiers returning is applied to those who have sustained grave injuries, bombs and the small but devastating improvised explosive devices (IEDs) being the main cause of very severe injury. These include loss of limbs, but also eviscerated abdomens, burst lungs and severe contamination. The reason for these 'unexpected survivors' coming through these severe bodily onslaughts is the high standard of medicine and nursing care in the field and the speed of the air rescue and transfer to the state-of-the-art field hospitals. The Times journalist's description of the work of these medical recovery teams[11] sums up the ethical aspect of these almost unbearable to think about cases:
>
>> These are the catastrophic injuries that the men and women of Task Force Dustoff deal with almost every day. (Starkey, 2010)
>
> He reports that these medical teams were averaging higher numbers of missions than in previous times, there being an average of 250 missions a month. In words which have their place in an ethics text book, Starkey describes how the doctors and nurses involved in these missions and at the field hospital live with the situation:
>
>> They cope through a mixture of courage, conscience and grim gallows humour, without which they claim they would go mad. (Starkey, 2010)
>
> The percentage of survivors is much increased by the system, making the ratio of dead to injured around 1:6. The ethical dilemma in all of this is described by one of the specialists on the US medical team. He told the journalist:
>
>> I've sent young soldiers home without any legs, terribly burnt, incapable of having children. I've kept them alive because it's my job. But I wonder, given the terrible extent of their wounds, whether it'd have been better if some of them hadn't made it. (Starkey, 2010)

---

[11]This is not an ethics of war discussion, but it should be noted that not all crews of these rescue helicopters have survived their missions.

The quality of the rescue service along with the need to move casualties out of the field hospitals in order to accommodate those coming in means that some soldiers returning to the UK will only regain consciousness when they arrive at Selly Oak's[12] intensive care unit.

The dilemma related by this field hospital surgeon raises the same moral issues as the ones that arise in the assisted-dying debates at the end of life. The central question is: 'When is it worth continuing with life?' It is an impossible question, one which McLean advises that we should not attempt to second-guess. But the obvious next question is: 'Who should decide?' The main thrust of the case, put forward by those arguing for the legal right to be assisted to die at a time of their choosing, is that the decision should rest with the person concerned. The ethical principle of best interests is a useful concept in this debate. The idea of best interests of the person concerned gives prime importance to 'value of the life for the person who must live it', as opposed to 'the value the person's life has for other persons' (Beauchamp and Childress, 2001: 103). The problems arise when the request to end life goes beyond the law when it requires action on the part of another person because withdrawal of treatment or cessation of ventilation is not relevant to the situation.

Physician-assisted Dying: The Ultimate Rights-based Choice

The question that has emerged from the end-of-life discussions among the health care professions and within society is whether there is a right to choose when and how one will die. Is this the ultimate rights-based ethics choice? Is it a demand too far that stretches the rights-based theory beyond what it is reasonable to expect? Or has it become a legitimate demand of 21st-century health care? The debates around this issue demonstrate how classic dilemmas that have ethical and legal dimensions can serve to illustrate the basic ethical principles which underpin our more mundane everyday moral choices. We can think about ethics for nursing and health care practice along a continuum from the basic everyday rights to personal care and nutrition through to the ultimate rights question: namely, the right to die at a time and in a manner of one's choosing.

Rights at both ends and along this continuum are not so clear cut as a continuum suggests. At the extreme end on the question of the right to die, society has

---

[12]Selly Oak Hospital in Birmingham is the specialist military hospital that receives casualties from war zones.

a view. The legal system in a liberal and democratic society is naturally cautious in drafting laws that have the potential for making some groups in society vulnerable. At the more basic end of the continuum, the seemingly simple matters of personal care and nutrition turn out to be, at times, bafflingly problematic. Recent experience[13] has shown that it is not always the case that safe and ethical practice, even in these most basic areas of need, is achieved. It is important to remember that the instances of bad care, appalling and horrible as they are, constitute a minority given the total scale of the health care service. A minority they may be, but importantly the problem, where it exists, seems to be systemic. The problems are rooted in the organisation and the practices have become institutionalised and seemingly beyond the reach of management.[14] The fact that the scandals of poor-quality care, and worse, are in a minority should not render us complacent. There is a moral imperative to establish and maintain in the NHS and private sector robust systems to regulate care and safeguard the public. In the doing of this, though, it is important not to cause unintended damage to the service and the staff, who are in the main doing a good job. There must be, in other words, room for professional judgement, for *phronesis* – Aristotle's practical wisdom and common sense (see Chapter 6). I cannot speak for Aristotle's day, but today common sense appears not to be that common!

It is clear that legal concerns dominate these developments in end-of-life care. If health care professionals are to take patient autonomy seriously, there needs to be a unified approach to end-of-life care which can satisfy professional and public expectations. There is understandable reluctance in governments to change the legal position vis-à-vis assisted dying. There are fears of rendering groups vulnerable and worries that a change in the law might prove to be a thin end of a wedge taking them into difficulties. It is important to have empirical research evidence available in ethical debate in order that we can be sure that the discussions of moral principles are engaged with the empirical reality, with how things are on the ground rather than being diverted by wedge-driven objections. For example, the research from the Netherlands provided evidence on which to evaluate objections frequently levelled at any proposed change in the law on assisted dying: Rietjens et al. (2009) published a paper entitled 'Two decades of research on euthanasia from the Netherlands. What have we learnt and what questions remain'. This title speaks for itself and the work provides some insights into the experience of euthanasia in the Netherlands and shows that some of the usual objections to euthanasia are unfounded. For example, there has been no 'slippery slope' experience, and physicians have followed the guidance in a large majority of cases.

---

[13]Mid Staffordshire NHS Trust failures of care and unnecessary deaths.

[14]The Francis Report (2013) on the Mid Staffordshire NHS Trust found 'a culture focused on doing the system's business, not that of the patients'. The challenge in the implementation of the Francis Report recommendations will be to change the organisational culture and the attitude of management.

Rights and Organ Donation

Organ donation is a good example of the importance of the social context in ethical debate. UK donor numbers are increasing. This is likely to be due to more families being asked and specialist nurses being employed to make the approach and explain to them the transplant programme and donor shortages. In fact, the UK has the highest number of people who are opposed to donating organs. Whilst one might suppose that what happens to a person's body after death is very much the business of that person, the family is approached for permission even though it is the case that there is no right in law for next of kin to exercise any rights in this respect. In spite of the legal position,[15] it is a matter of custom and practice that doctors approach the family for permission to use the organs, and the result is that potential donors are lost. This is rather like overriding a person's will and, whilst a will might be contested, there is a general presumption that what a person willed in life should come about after their death. It is the last opportunity to show respect for the dead.

The ethical argument for allowing organ donation, especially if the deceased has expressed that wish, rests on both non-maleficence and beneficence for the donor and recipient respectively. Once there is no longer a possibility of life for the potential donor, the question of non-maleficence does not arise for no harm can be done. The overwhelming case is for beneficence with regard to the recipient of the organ. This argument is compelling and is evidenced, to an extent, in the fact that some countries uphold a policy of opt-out for organ donation. In other words, the presumption is that someone would want to donate and if not they have the right to register an opt-out choice. Mason and Laurie (2011: 551) in their discussion note that in Italy and in Spain, where there is a 'contracting out model' (opt out) in operation, there is 'a power of veto is still vested in the next of kin'.

Rights-based ethical theory is perhaps the most useful of the ethical theories when it comes to considering the ethical issues in organ donation. It might also be the case that more emphasis on rights and less on sentiment would best serve justice in the transplant service – more Kantian than 'Smithian categorical imperative' in this case. Also if we consider the social and cultural context in which organ donation takes place, it seems to me that there are other ways of approaching the practical business of obtaining organs. The practice would change for the better, in terms of success in obtaining organs, if the next of kin could be helped to see through the wishes of their deceased relative rather than being asked for their permission. There is an analogy here with the way that the post-mortem process is organised. In the case of post-mortem the next of kin have no veto, as the performing of a post-mortem is a requirement of law. There must exist an accompanying social process which organises the post-mortem whilst keeping the next of kin informed. There may be lessons there for the health service and its transplant service which would assist in bringing about a change in the culture whereby the priority is having a sufficient supply of

---

[15]There is no legal right of the next of kin to have a veto on the matter of organ donation. Indeed, the body after death does not 'belong' to anyone, even to the deceased.

organs and a climate in which citizens are content to play their part. This is an example of society's role in ethical debate.

The concerns of the organ transplant service are clearly not mainstream. However, these problems and the discussion of possible solutions serve as an example of the interdependency of society and the health service. The right that citizens have to safe and effective health care is matched by their duty to engage as members of society and to contribute as a matter of public duty in various ways: for instance, by participation in research, to take part in drug trials when invited to do so and to enrol as blood and organ donors. At a more everyday level, members of society have an obligation to participate in public health measures for the common good. Public health is an area of health care where individualism and autonomy cannot be the main ethical principles underlying practice. Public health involves us as individuals, but only in the sense of individuals as members of the wider group. Herd immunity that is required for protection against disease is not a matter of individual choice, it is a matter of collective responsibility. It is a classic example of the limits to rights.

- Rights are justifiable claims, legal or moral, that individuals can make upon others or upon society.
- Patients have a right to competent safe treatment. A competent adult patient can refuse any treatment as of right.
- The unintended consequences of risk management can result in the infringement of patients' rights.

9

Virtue Ethics and Professional Regulation

Hamlet: What's the news?
Rosencrantz: None my Lord, but that the world's grown honest.

Shakespeare. c.1600, *Hamlet*, II, ii

Virtue ethics is an increasingly popular approach to ethical discussion in nursing and health care. The focus is upon the person of the practitioner and their virtues: integrity, competence, wisdom, kindness and so on. Virtue ethics focuses on the individual practitioner and their attributes, the idea being to think in terms of what constitutes the virtuous practitioner. The professional code and the underlying principles of nursing practice are important, but when an individual practitioner does not behave in line with ethical codes there are problems, potentially serious ones. The focus on the individual is appropriate when it comes to ethics for practice because the quality of nursing care comes down in the end to the performance of each nurse day in and day out.

Virtue ethics has a rather quaint ring about it. It somehow conjures up the idea of the virtuous woman and sounds rather too 19th-century for our purposes. We are concerned with ethics for practice in the 21st century, having thrown off the image of an all-female profession working very much in the shadow of medicine. We have long since nudged aside the idea of etiquette in favour of ethics for practice. However, it would be a mistake to be put off by a label. As it happens, virtue ethics goes all the way back to ancient Greece and Aristotle (384–322 BC) and his idea of virtue ethics. Aristotle taught about virtues in connection with his question 'What is the good life?'. The questions that follow from this are: 'What is the right thing to do?', 'How should I behave?'. These are important questions for nursing practice.

Virtue ethics is one of the various approaches to ethics for practice that we find in nursing and medical ethics texts. It is said to be attractive to health care professionals because of its focus upon the individual professional: that is, on the person.

The emphasis upon competency based training in the health care professions is not without its difficulties but it fits well with virtue ethics because it focuses upon the individual practitioner. It is perhaps not surprising that Aristotle is so popular all these years on when we know that much of the work that we have access to is essentially his teaching notes. As Barnes[1] puts it:

> Aristotle's treatises, as we have them, all stem from the lecture courses on philosophical and scientific subjects which he gave during his long teaching career – they are his lecture notes. (in Thomson, 1976: 15)

Barnes adds that:

> [t]he ancient editors doubtless indulged in ordering and polishing, but what we have here before us is essentially what Aristotle had on the lectern in front of him when he addressed his pupils. (in Thomson, 1976: 15)

Aristotle's body of work is extensive. We are concerned here with a small part of his work on ethics, specifically his work on virtue. We have already noted that the there are similarities between what we now call 'competencies' and Aristotle's notion of virtue.

The problem with the presentation of various ethical theories as if they are in opposition to one another is that it suggests that there must be one best theory. The impression that can be gained on coming to ethical theories for the first time is perhaps that it has to be one theory or another, utilitarianism or deontology, rights-based ethics or respect for persons, and the one that trumps the others is the one to follow, whereas in fact they can complement one another. Utilitarianism, roughly speaking, focuses on the majority and leaves out the minority. Rationing a health care budget along utilitarian lines would leave out minority needs, neo-natal intensive care, for example, or IVF. A focus on the individual, respect for a person's autonomy, takes a different viewpoint, one where individuals count. It is more a matter of emphasis and perspective and a consideration of the various arguments helps to arrive at a balanced view. Rationing in terms of allocation of budgets involves decisions about what takes priority, where resources are directed. Sometimes these decisions involve financial sums of such a magnitude that it is difficult to really make sense of them, or at least to relate them to our own experience of practice. If we think about it in terms of how we organise our time on a ward, how we decide where to spend time, we can get some feel for rationing. Do we leave some people out of our calculation because they are less in need of attention than others? Do we have to spread ourselves evenly in the name of fairness? These small decisions that rely on individual judgement give us some practical idea of what it is to ration care.

---

[1]Jonathan Barnes wrote the introduction in J.A.K. Thomson's (1976) translation, *The Ethics of Aristotle – The Nicomachean Ethics*.

A student nurse and a health care assistant (HCA) on a busy surgical ward have been allocated a small number of patients. The charge nurse has selected a group with differing levels of dependency so that it should be possible to balance their needs and accomplish the care for the morning. The student finds it difficult to manage the very demanding requests from one patient. The patient, a young woman, was expected to be independent and able to get to the bathroom and day room without assistance, but she constantly asked for help, saying that she was tired. The student found it hard to know whether this was so, and in any case did not feel that she should judge her and so helped. This, of course, meant that the other patients, who were dependent, were left for longer periods than was desirable. Also as she was working with the HCA for the patients who required two members of staff to lift, she was causing misuse of her time too.

In this example it comes down to an individual trying to ration their time in a fair way, and such a decision probably has more to do with judgement and a sense of fairness than a utilitarian calculation.

Virtue Ethics

The advantage that the virtue ethics approach has is that it focuses on the competence and integrity of the practitioner, or in the moral philosopher's language 'the moral agent'. This approach avoids some of the problem of feeling the need to set theory against theory. Virtue ethics also sits well with Aristotle's work; indeed, some would go so far as to say that Aristotle was a kind of virtue ethicist. Virtue ethics perhaps offers a middle ground between the overly subjective conscience and the abstract objectivity of some of the less immediately practical moral theories. Virtue ethics has certainly been given prominence recently in ethics texts in health care.

In *The Nicomachean Ethics* (Thomson, 1976), Aristotle talks of two kinds of virtue that are complementary. We should note that in ancient Greek 'virtue' meant *an excellence*, what we would now call a 'competence'. These two types of virtues or competencies Aristotle calls the 'intellectual' and the 'moral' virtues. Aristotle says that both kinds of virtue are needed for an individual to be able to decide how to act in a morally acceptable way, morally appropriate and appropriate to the situation. The *intellectual* virtues involve knowledge and competence for decision making and problem solving. So for nursing practice, we are talking about the biomedical and the psychosocial knowledge bases of the discipline. The *moral* virtues, on the other hand, have to do with the character that Aristotle thought to be necessary for reliable and effective action. Aristotle thought that there had to be a balance between these two kinds of virtue for people to act in moral ways. Already we can see that the idea of virtue, or excellence, is very close to the competencies around which education programmes of preparation for nursing and the other health professions organise the curriculum.

Aristotle's intellectual or theoretical virtues include relevant scientific knowledge, technical skill, intelligence, insight, resourcefulness, discriminatory judgement and practical wisdom. The moral virtues relate to character and include honesty, courage, integrity, loyalty, temperance, justice, generosity and magnanimity. If we consider these listings we can see that the balance of virtues that Aristotle deemed to be necessary – the intellectual and the moral virtues – essentially have to do with wisdom and justice. In Aristotle's *Nicomachean Ethics* he defines what he calls *phronesis* as 'practical wisdom, prudence and common sense'. Setting these virtues down in total does rather suggest that the nurse has to be some kind of paragon. They are included for the sake of completeness. The idea of a virtuous person includes the main virtues, but also it carries the idea of a decent, honest and competent practitioner.

Being a virtuous person in Aristotle's day involved being excellent at doing something. If we transfer this idea to the practice of nursing, we are looking at a nurse who is able to make decisions that draw on knowledge and good judgement. And the care resulting from these decisions would be carried out in a caring way with respect for the patient's autonomy and rights to confidentiality. The idea of *phronesis* sits well with this idea of the virtuous practitioner because we can think of an ethical practitioner as one who draws upon these virtues in order to arrive at clinical decisions that are based on knowledge and made with regard to the circumstances and emotional aspects of the case. One of Aristotle's ideas that is useful when we think about ethics for nursing practice is his writing about habituation. He says that 'moral virtues, like crafts, are acquired by practice and habituation' (Book II, 1103a14–b1). The more we do something, the better we become at doing it.

Aristotle's thesis is that ethical virtues are instilled in people by habit; they are not automatically in us by nature. His idea was that virtues, or states of character, are acquired by undertaking the virtuous acts in the same way that one would do it if one already had that virtue, or as Aristotle puts it, already had that 'state of character'. It might be thought that virtue ethics, with its focus on the attributes of the moral agent that is the individual practitioner, is in danger of taking us back into the difficulties thrown up by a reliance upon individual consciences as a guide to action. However, virtue ethics has the merit that it brings to our attention the fact that the quality of the actions of individuals depends upon the integrity and competence of the individual. Virtue ethics focuses on the moral agent: for our purposes this means the individual practitioner. This is exactly the focus of the statutory regulatory bodies when they set up the procedures for the production and maintenance of a professional register. The links between virtue ethics and the requirements of professional regulation are clear. For those who enjoy sociological analysis, the fit is perfect: if your source of satisfaction lies elsewhere, no matter, because the relevance can still be appreciated.

Campbell et al. focus on the qualities of moral sensitivity and integrity in their discussion of virtue ethics and say that:

> we must ask what it is to be a person of sensitivity and integrity. We might suggest that it is to be a 'person of sound character'. This claim brings us close to what is called virtue theory, and is reminiscent of Hume's person of sound sentiment.

> According to virtue theory, it is character that is the focus of moral concern, and someone who shows virtues such as kindness, generosity, respect for persons, honesty and compassion will be the model of moral conduct. (2005: 8)

Clearly the virtue ethics approach amounts to more than leaving the question of ethics to the good sense and judgement of professionals. This is not to say that we should be naturally suspicious of health care professionals. However, what we need is, as Campbell et al. put it:

> to devise a conception of virtuous practice that does not suggest that a doctor or nurse can dictate what ought to happen to other people. (2005: 8)

In other words, whilst it is the individual professional that needs to be a person of integrity, honesty, knowledgeable and so on, the scrutiny of the professions is a public matter. The statutory regulation of the health care professions is a transparent, robust and public process.

Ethic of Care and Virtue Ethics

Within the writings on nursing ethics in the 1980s and 1990s there emerged what was called 'the ethics of care' (sometimes the 'ethic' of care) (Larrabee, 1993), which focused on the activity of caring for people. The ethic of care addresses the issues that arise in the business of caring for people – nursing's business. Nursing's legacy of being in a subordinate relationship to a dominant medical profession was further impetus to the desire by nurses to articulate a unique body of knowledge for nursing and to develop an area of practice which nursing can claim as its own. As part of this quest, nursing ethics texts have tended to follow two particular themes that medical ethics texts were not dealing with: these are the ethics of care and advocacy, and they tend to be presented as nursing's business.[2]

The ethic of care, or certainly its popularity, owes much to the work of Carol Gilligan. Her book *In a Different Voice: Psychological Theory and Women's Development* (1982) presented a challenge to Kohlberg's (1981) analysis of moral reasoning by suggesting that there were gendered differences in approach to moral reasoning. In studying the moral reasoning processes that girls use, Gilligan (1982) in her analysis offered an ethic of care which she contrasted with the ethic of justice and rights. Kohlberg, on the basis of his study of boys' moral development, had argued that boys employed ideas of justice and rights in arriving at moral judgements. Writers in the field of nursing ethics seized on Gilligan's work as a useful means of furthering nursing's professionalising project, staking out and developing a distinctive role, which would be different from that of medicine.

---

[2] For further discussion, see Melia (2004).

Gilligan makes a clear distinction between *caring* and *justice* as two moral perspectives employed in making moral judgements. In playground disputes, boys go to the rules of the game and demand justice. In a similar situation, girls take more notice of how everyone feels and look for compromise and to please everyone. Caring emphasises a character trait of the practitioner, hence the link to virtue ethics. Justice is a more objective principle, one of the four put forward by Beauchamp and Childress as it happens. An understanding of Gilligan's position on an ethic of care is best expressed in her rejoinder to those whom she thought had misunderstood her, or certainly misrepresented her work. In 1993 Gilligan, in a comment on reactions to her earlier work (1982), argued that she had been misrepresented by many who take the gender thesis too far and too literally when they made the link between male and justice and female and caring. The 'different voice', she notes, 'is identified not by gender but by theme'. She describes two moral perspectives, *care* and *justice*, that she says:

> organize both thinking and feelings and empower the self to take different kinds of action in public as well as private life. (1993: 209)

Gilligan says that the title of her book was deliberate: it reads, she reminds us, 'in a different voice', not 'in a woman's voice' (Gilligan, in Larrabee, 1993: 209).

Campbell et al. say that there are similarities between the *ethics of care* and *virtue ethics*, and they note that:

> it [ethics of care] has grown up in nursing ethics where the problems of power hierarchies, the role of women, and the actual experience of tending to people's needs have combined to yield a very different perspective on the ethical situation from that traditionally found in books of medical ethics. (2005: 15)

Campbell et al. go further when they say that the ethic of care is in some ways a virtue theory,

> in that it privileges the judgement of those who have actually been involved in the morally challenging situations under discussion, and struggled to cope with the experiences they found there. What it has added is not a mere substitution of the concept of care for concepts like autonomy and beneficence, but rather a sensitive appreciation of practical needs, caring responses to those needs, and the wisdom resulting from such encounters. (2005: 15–16)

Ethics of care has clear links with virtue ethics because it focuses upon the activity of caring and therefore on the professional's activity, and style of practice. Following Campbell et al., we might say that this distinction is between *virtue theory* and *justice*.

Virtue ethics is in many ways a more inclusive theory than the ethics of care, as the latter tends to separate nursing from the wider health care team. This, I would argue, is possibly because nursing was too concerned to be seen to be different from medicine, to be a profession in its own right. In staking out its territory and designating care as the distinctive work of nursing, medicine was, intentionally or otherwise, cast in the role of 'cure'. Clearly it is medicine's business to cure and treat appropriately when cure is not an option. But when 'cure' is mentioned in nursing texts in order to distinguish 'care' as 'nursing's business', the term 'cure' has a slightly pejorative hint about it. The facts of the matter are that the medical curriculum contains a good deal about care, and to suggest that care does not come along with the cure remit is plain silly. This division of health care work is a rather simplistic split, an artificial distinction between care and cure that focuses too much upon the differences, which is not helpful for teamwork.

The ethic of care might be said to have been overtaken by virtue ethics, which is less exclusionary and so more conducive to teamwork, and perhaps more importantly paves the way for a broader approach to ethics for health care practice.

Professional Regulation

A profession has to have its own integrity and to be able to demonstrate this to the public. Professional regulation is essentially about trust and trustworthiness. Occupations which lay claim to professional status and thereby enjoy a privileged position in the hierarchy of occupations have mechanisms in place for their regulation. Self-regulation is part of the professional culture in which a profession has control over its practice and practitioners. Beyond this there has to be some independent oversight of the regulation and assurance for the public that the professions are acting in the interests of society and not in their own self-interest. One of the hallmarks of a profession is that it operates in an altruistic way and not primarily for profit. In exchange for this altruism in the approach to their work, professions are granted a certain amount of freedom to pursue their mission with little unnecessary interference.

The balance between professional freedom and public protection is the concern of professional regulation. If the balance tips towards too much regulation and 'red tape' and the regulatory process is too restrictive and prescriptive, the more wide-reaching problem is that these regulatory constraints might undermine professionalism and professional autonomy. In the longer run, this might do harm in terms of recruitment to the profession and in turn this could present difficulties in terms of retention of nurses already in the profession.

The initiatives that follow hard on the heels of inquiries into poor standards of care have on occasion been 'prescribed' on a national basis, from central government, even the Prime Minister's office rather than the Department of Health. For example, following the Mid Staffordshire Inquiry the idea that patients should be asked, on an hourly basis, if they were in need of anything came from the Prime Minister. The idea,

(Continued)

(Continued)

appropriately tailored to the situation, is not in itself a bad one. However, it is a very long-standing part of nursing care and for many charge nurses (indeed, many qualified nurses) it would be part of their professional repertoire. Blanket instruction to do the obvious has its consequences, and like many routinised activities, the point can be lost and no gain had.

This example has caused much debate and as with many seemingly good ideas it is not easy to argue against without sounding as if patient care is not the main concern. This 'intentional rounding' is not going to be appropriate for every situation. Random good ideas do not, in the longer run, help in situations that have arisen as a result of a complex of institutional and organisational factors which individuals have failed to overcome. The Mid Staffordshire scandal is a case in point. Simple solutions are rather like financial bargains, where if the price looks too good to be true, it probably is. If a solution appears to be simple, it is probably too simple to be a match for the problem.

If we go back to the ideas of Chapter 5 and think about these in terms of 'practical reason' and the idea that 'reasons that are justifying reasons have a bearing on how one decides to act' (MacCormick, 2008: 12), we might want to consider the merits of blanket instructions issued to cover both those who perhaps are in need of some guidance and those who clearly are not.

Part of the ethics for nursing practice is about being able to think plans through, employing the virtues as outlined from Aristotle's work, to arrive at well considered approaches to practice which will serve patients' best interests. It is highly likely that it was this kind generalised edict that led to the bizarre situation recounted in Chapter 3, where the nurse woke a patient up 'at four in the morning!' to ask her what she would like for lunch.

The point is that if professional judgement is overridden in a wholesale way, the resultant effect on practice is unpredictable. The nature of professional practice includes decision making and a presumption of clinical competence. Random interference and additional paperwork along with a judgemental attitude from the centre erodes professionalism and does not necessarily bode well for patient care. If we are going to take ethics for practice seriously, we have to be prepared to think these kinds of issues through and not simply accept that there is an easy answer to problems. If an immediate response is thought to be helpful, there is no reason not to go along with it, but in the longer run these matters have to be thought through and discussed. The discussion should include all aspects of care and its organisation and not least the ethical principles upon which it rests. This approach is especially apt if the problem, as in the Mid Staffordshire case, seems to be a basic one – food out of reach, basic needs neglected. The question has to be, 'How have we arrived at this situation?' It is a question that nurses should be prepared to ask themselves, to return to the basic ethical principles and ask 'How has it come to this?' and 'How do we sort it out?'. Ethical debate is a practical matter, sorting it out is a practical solution. The gap between how things are and how they ought to be is a long-standing question for ethics.

Nursing and Midwifery Council

We conclude this chapter with a brief look at nursing's statutory regulatory body.

Nursing is a statutorily regulated profession: that is to say, the regulation takes its authority from an Act of Parliament (Nurses, Midwives and Health Visitors Act, 1997). The Nursing and Midwifery Council (NMC) oversees the work of registered nurses and sets the standards that the universities running education programmes for nurses, midwives and health visitors must meet. The work of the NMC is essentially about the protection of the public. Its strapline on all publications is: 'Protecting the public through professional standards.'

There are two main ways in which the regulatory body ensures safe and competent practice: first, through the professional register that governs who is entitled to be recognised in law as a practitioner; and second, by setting and maintaining standards. The NMC is also the route through which alleged professional misconduct is judged.

The NMC maintains a register of nurses, midwives and health visitors. Those entered on the register must reach the required standards of the professional education for the part of the register on which their name appears. The NMC sets the standards that are required to be met by those on the register. The programmes of education are based in the universities and work in partnership with the NHS Trusts and validated by the NMC to produce graduates whose degrees make them eligible to apply to have their name entered on the register. In this way both the individual practitioner and the programmes of education are under the regulatory gaze of the NMC. Both of these functions are clearly large and complex undertakings.

There are three parts to the register, namely, nurses, midwives and specialist community public health nurses. Health visitors continue to have separate registration and representation in the NMC, but appear on the register listed as 'specialist community public health nurse'.[3] The essential functions of the NMC are:

- keeping the register of members admitted to practice;
- determining the standards of education and learning for admission to practise;
- giving guidance about standards of conduct and performance; and
- administering procedures relating to misconduct, unfitness to practise and similar matters.

The Council for Healthcare Regulatory Excellence (CHRE), now known as the Professional Standards Authority for Helath and Social Care, is the body that

---

[3] In 2002 the new profession of Specialist Community Public Health Nurse was created and comes under the NMC regulation.

oversees the regulatory bodies of all the health care professions. It was set up in 2002 following the passing of the National Health Service Reform and Health Care Professionals Act (2002). The body was established after the Kennedy Report (Bristol Royal Infirmary Inquiry, 2001) into the children's heart surgery at the Bristol Royal Infirmary. This report followed the inquiry into the higher number of deaths following surgery than should be expected. The competence of the surgeons involved was questioned. This is an example of the public scrutiny of health care practitioners.

The CHRE exists to provide a body which overarches the professions' regulatory bodies, and its remit is to protect and promote the interests of patients and the public in general.

The Council produced a report on the NMC following complaints that the NMC was not fulfilling its purpose and obligations, including a back-log of cases. The CHRE report noted serious problems with the governance and culture of the NMC. This led to reorganisation and change of senior members of the NMC. Changes in CHRE itself were suggested following the Department of Health and Chief Medical Officer's review of the whole business of professional regulation.

All of this may seem to be administrative detail that has no place in a book about ethics for practice. It is, however, an illustration of the complexity of regulation and the protection of the public. The legal system has its checks and balances, higher courts to which there is a system of appeal and judicial review where application can be made to a High Court for a judicial or administrative decision to be reviewed and a 'declaration' (a ruling setting out the legal position) made. We see that the professional regulatory system also has its checks and overseeing bodies which have the power to make changes in the system when it is deemed to be failing.

The point of interest here is that professional regulation is crucial to the safe functioning of health care services and the protection of the public. It is also a very complicated business, and large organisations can have difficulties which are more than technical or legal matters. Large organisations such as the health service have to consider integrity, ethics and culture. We saw in Chapter 3 the importance of understanding the context within which ethical issues arise. Culture is very much an area of study for sociologists and it is notable that the Francis Report (2013) specifically mentioned that one of the problems at Mid Staffordshire was the culture that had developed which gave more importance to targets and gaining Foundation Trust status for the hospital than it did to the quality of patient care.

Code of Conduct

The NMC code of professional conduct[4] is articulated in the document *The Code: Standards of Conduct, Performance and Ethics for Nurses and Midwives*, published

---

[4]See www.nmc-uk.org. There is also guidance for students in the NMC (2011) publication.

in 2008; it was redesigned in 2010 but the content remains the same. There are three main points in the Code that are central to our discussion of virtue ethics:

- Make care of people your first concern, treating them as individuals and respecting their dignity.
- As a professional, you are personally accountable for actions and omissions in your practice and must always be able to justify your decisions.
- You must always act lawfully, whether those laws relate to your professional practice or personal life.

The NMC Code is not enforceable in law but it is based on the principles that the law embraces, and it has the power to remove names from the register in the event of professional misconduct. The Code is used by the committees concerned with professional misconduct. The Conduct and Competence Committee of the NMC[5] is concerned with fitness to practise. The standard of proof required in these proceedings is the 'balance of probabilities', which is the same as in civil law cases (the criminal law standard is 'beyond reasonable doubt').

The Code requires that all nurses, midwives and health visitors practise within an ethical framework. The basic principles of the code centre upon respect for the patients and clients. The Code stresses that practitioners must recognise their moral obligations and the need to accept personal responsibility for their own ethical choices, within specific situations, based on their own professional judgement. In making such choices, practitioners must be aware of, and adhere to, legal as well as professional requirements. Nurses are accountable for their actions; this accountability is to the patient, the public, the NMC and the employing authority.

Personal and Professional Morals

In complex societies where there are many faith groups and those with no religious affiliation and agnostics and atheists living alongside each other, the question of the place of religion in public life is a not an easy one. The landmark case of Dr Leonard Arthur,[6] which concerned the non-treatment of a newborn and the eventual charging of the paediatrician with murder following a high-profile trial in the criminal court in England in 1981, is a good example. The case raised many legal questions at the time concerning what was described as the 'selective non-treatment of the

---

[5]See Dimond (2011), Chapter 11, for a discussion of details of the powers of the Fitness to Practise Committee. Dimond (2011) is an excellent reference work and is included here so that this discussion of ethics does not become overly burdened with disciplinary procedure and the mechanics of regulation.

[6]R v. Arthur (1981) 12 BMLR 1.

newborn' and the 'withholding of the means of survival from mentally handicapped[7] infants' (Mason and Laurie, 2011: 475).

> Leonard Arthur, a consultant paediatrician, was tried for the murder of a baby with Down's syndrome. The condition was initially thought to be uncomplicated. The parents were distressed by the baby's condition and had expressed a wish that efforts should not be made to prolong the baby's life. Dr Arthur wrote in the notes, 'The parents do not wish him to survive; nursing care only.' He prescribed sedation to relieve the baby's distress and the baby died four days later. A member of Life working in the hospital contacted the police and alleged that the baby had been drugged and left to die. Dr Arthur was charged with murder. The charge was reduced to attempted murder following the autopsy medical evidence that the baby also had physical abnormalities. Throughout the trial the prosecution conceded that Dr Arthur's motives were of the highest order, acting as he saw in the interests of the family and the baby; however, they maintained that doctors were not above the law. Expert medical witnesses endorsed Dr Arthur's view and he was acquitted.

Mason and Laurie also note that Dr Arthur's actions are very unlikely to be condoned today. They see the case as, in their words,

> an example of the dangers of extrapolating the concept of 'futility' to one of an obligation not to treat in the face of parental pressure. (2011: 480)

Following what Mason and Laurie describe as a 'cultural shift ... away from medical paternalism towards parental autonomy', they note that there have been:

> marked changes in judicial attitudes towards the care of patients in extreme and harrowing conditions such as persistent vegetative state or neuro-degenerative disorders. (2011: 475)

All of these matters are of concern for nursing practice because nurses will be involved in the care of the infants in such situations, however the legal cases play out. But our interest in the Arthur case in the context of this chapter lies in the fact that it was alleged that it was a member of the nursing staff, who also belonged to a pro-life activist group, who informed the police, leading to the court case. The fact

---

[7]'Handicapped' was the terminology of the 1980s and was regarded as an improvement upon earlier terms for mental disability such as 'imbecile', 'feeble-minded' and worse. Today we say 'learning disability', a term which in my view is misleading as it suggests that a remedy lies in education and does not convey the severity of the disability in many cases. In trying to avoid any stigma in a label it conveys it in an inverse fashion. 'Mental disability' would be a more accurate term and one on equal footing with 'physical disability'.

that there was a high-profile criminal prosecution drew public attention to the question of non-treatment of neonates, which was very much an aim of the activists.

The important questions are: 'Can professionals remain neutral?', 'Are there occasions when nurses should take up causes because the public would take more notice of a professional viewpoint?' and 'Should the plight of individual patients be used to make political points?'.

In the Arthur case, the parents were unaware of the fact that they were being observed by a member of staff who espoused a cause which took exception to their decisions. The member of the pro-life group might have thought that her action was prompted by a concern for what she regarded as an infringement of the infant's right to live. It might be argued that the nurse had in mind more concern for the general cause of the pro-life organisation than she had for the individual rights and needs of the baby in question. After all, Dr Arthur had taken the decision in consultation with the parents and with the approval of the nursing staff directly involved in the care.

An increasingly well informed public, the availability of information on the Internet and a culture that encourages individualism means that the health service has to contend with the views of well informed patients and lobby groups. How reasonable is it for nurses to bring their private views into the workplace? In the Arthur case, where the police were involved, the nurse was using her position in the hospital and the fact that she was privy to information about the baby's care to further the cause of the pro-life group.

There are, of course, good reasons for wanting to have people in the health care professions who are prepared to make moral stands and to accept that there is a moral dimension to their work. It is not necessarily the case that we need activists on particular matters, and there has to be a limit to what is deemed to be a reasonable expression of opinion and what goes a step too far and becomes a misuse of a position of privilege.

The reason that there is a professional code is that it can be shared by members of the profession, and so the public can be assured that there is an agreed standard and set of principles – rules of the game, if you like – that everyone is playing by regardless of their personal morality. One of the main functions of a code of professional conduct is precisely this matter of informing the public of our mission and guiding principles – running the profession's values up the flagpole, as it were.

The codes of conduct of regulated professions can at times be inflexible and produce odd results.

For example, a community nurse was on duty when she came upon a child whom she thought was somewhere between three and five years old. The child was getting in and out of a car which was parked near shops on a busy road. Seeing that the child was unaware of the dangers of playing in the road, she waited with the child for a short while, saw no adult, and decided it was best to take the child with her to her patient

(Continued)

(Continued)

'literally just round the corner'. She left a note with her mobile number on the car windscreen where the child was playing. The note said that the community nurse had the child, and to 'phone'. Within two minutes, according to the press report, the nurse was 'phoned by the father who had been longer than he intended away from his car. He was apparently very grateful to the nurse for keeping his child safe.'

The nurse then informed her practice's team leader; according to the press she says that making this call was the 'worst mistake' of her life. The police were soon involved, she was suspended and the NMC investigated and suspended the nurse for six months, and beyond that the NMC imposed an 18-month period during which she would have conditions imposed on her practice. The basis of all this was 'displaying serious failings in child protection'. The NMC report states that the nurse's actions and behaviour 'breached the standards expected of a registered nurse and are a serious departure from good practice'. It goes on to say that she 'has not acknowledged the potential risks her actions could have had and the distress she could have caused to the child's parents'.

The nurse is taking the case to law. Her view is that she was in uniform and as far as she was concerned following the Code, which puts care of people as a priority. Her lawyer is confident of a positive outcome.

Without all the details it is not possible to judge a case. However, on the face of it this does seem to be a case of over-reaction on the part of the NMC – sledgehammers and nuts come to mind. The nurse made a decision at the time when she had a patient expecting her visit, she was in uniform and so felt that she could be trusted, and she left her contact number. She did not want to leave the child she had come upon in the dangerous busy road. The NMC took a principled view and considered the possible consequences. As it happens in this case, according to the press reports, the father was grateful and apologetic. The outcome was good: having left his child for longer than he had intended, the father was reunited with him in a matter of minutes and had no complaints, and he was indeed grateful to the nurse for her action.

The fact that the nurse saw fit to report this to her team leader is of interest, a decision we might question as she eventually did. One might argue that a professional nurse should be allowed to come to her own decisions in a case such as this – it certainly would be difficult to draw up detailed protocols for such an event. The NMC therefore fell back on principles and made, in my personal view, rather a meal of it. Readers may take a different view and employ what is often called the 'wedge' argument – as in thin end of – whereby the possible consequences of one's actions are taken into account in determining how to act. This example demonstrates the difficulty of deciding what to do. It could be said to be a dilemma, whereby one principle is compromised if one action is taken and another if a different decision is taken. The nurse chose to protect the child, at the risk of his parent's distress. Ironically, in so doing she was disciplined in the name of child protection.

This case points up the fact that individual professional views, the law, tribunals and professional regulatory bodies may all come to different conclusions on the case and the outcome in terms of registration. This investigation, and others like it, demonstrate that underlying nursing practice there are the virtues of moral judgement and trust in operation. This trust is required if the professional–patient relationship is going to work. The link between virtue ethics and professional regulation is similar to the link between a moral judgement and the enshrinement of that judgement in law, as we saw in the 'snail in the bottle' case which gave rise to the important concept of the duty of care, which underpins the laws of negligence. In both cases, professional regulation and the law, they are difficult to bring into alignment with the moral position. In the case of regulation, it is easy enough to articulate what we want from nurses, but less easy to regulate this, less easy to formulate the regulatory requirements.

A Matter of Balance

It is often the case that a moral argument can be made to support a clinical policy or decision. For example, the debates about the options that people have at the end of life are complex. One thing is clear: people hold strong views on the matter. The moral case for physician-assisted death can be made to the satisfaction of those who defend the right of an individual to have control over their life. Even if this were a universally held view, the task of turning the moral right into one that will stand up in law is a more difficult matter. All the consequences intended and unintended, known and unknown, are generally sufficient to deter law makers from decriminalising the assisting of a suicide. There are similar difficulties when it comes to enshrining, in professional regulation requirements, what expectations we might reasonably have of virtuous practice. The best we have are competencies and self-declarations of fitness to practise, both physical and moral. Competencies are, remember, close to Aristotle's idea of virtue, meaning an excellence. This brings us back to the question of the trustworthiness of individuals. Self-declarations and confirmation of the moral standing of a practitioner do not amount to much of a guarantee without the trust in the individual upon which they rest.

There are limits to what regulation can achieve in terms of a safe and competent workforce in health care. Post-Shipman[8] (see Chapter 3) there has been a shift in emphasis in public debates on professions which now focus more on character and the screening-out of criminals and less on professionally oriented regulation of competencies. Given the fact that professional regulation is about protection of the public, and that Shipman and the various other public scandals shook faith in the health care sector, this shift is perhaps to be expected. It should, though, be remembered that there is no such thing as 'risk-free', and if those drawing up professional

---

[8]See www.the-shipman-inquiry.org.uk.

standards have this as a goal, then there are likely to be unintended consequences which may leave the professionals with less discretion and more minded to avoid difficult decisions. Defensive practice may be superficially safe but it is not necessarily in the best interests of patients. The desired balance would be to produce a health service staffed by professionals who have some hand in drawing up the moral code by which they operate. Professional codes can be influential in the shaping of the law that affects the practice of health care.

Ultimately it comes down to trust in individual practitioners. Of course we need regulation, but there is a danger in an over-burdensome system of regulation, where attention to documentation and procedure predominates, that professional judgement is nudged aside in favour of rules and protocol. Knowing when to deviate from a rule can be important. Finally, it is well to remember that we are always in danger of undermining professional judgement and discretion by the use of too many sticks and the wrong carrot.

- Virtue ethics focuses on the individual practitioner and their attributes. The idea is to think in terms of what constitutes the virtuous practitioner.
- Enshrining in professional regulation requirements the expectations of virtuous practice is not easy: the best we have are competencies and self-declarations of fitness to practise, both physical and moral.
- Virtue ethics might be said to have overtaken the ethic of care. Virtue ethics is more inclusive and so conducive to teamwork.

10

Concluding Thoughts

If one does not know to which port one is sailing no wind is favourable.

Seneca, c.4BC–65 AD

The task of this short chapter is to draw together the main themes that permeate this discussion of ethics for nursing and health care practice. Two central ideas running through the discussion are *trust* and *judgement*, ideas that encompass the business of ethics for nursing and health care practice which ultimately comes down to reasoning out the solutions to the moral questions that arise.

Trust encompasses patients' trust in professionals and the trust that professionals have in each other and in their employing authorities. Nurses and other professionals in health care must be free to use their professional knowledge to make professional judgements. This evidence base for practice comes from the professions: it cannot be supplied by managers, nor by politicians. In the end it comes down to the fact that patients are in the hands of health care professionals, and patients have to rely on the integrity and good moral judgement of these professionals.

Aristotle's idea of *phronesis*, which means 'practical wisdom' and includes notions of 'prudence' and 'common sense', is as the name suggests, a very practical approach to decision making. Practical wisdom is employed in making judgements in health care and draws upon the factual, legal and the emotional aspects of the case. The moral aspect of health care is an integral part of the clinical judgements which are made every day. Professional ethical codes offer practitioners some guidance as to their actions, but a judgement is called for when making decisions. Judgement is required in order to answer the central practical question in the management of patient care: 'What to do now?' An important part of the Aristotelian idea of practical wisdom was the need to take account of the particular situation in order to arrive at the best answer in that circumstance. Aristotle's practical wisdom is similar to what we recognise today in professional clinical judgement in so far as we may set out with a clear principle-based theoretical view of what is the right thing to do, but circumstances may cause us to adjust and negotiate towards a better solution for the particular case.

We have seen from MacCormick's work on *Practical Reason in Law and Morality* (2008) that the process of practical reason is similar whether the intention is to arrive at a legal or a clinical judgement. The moral element has to be included in the reasoning. Adam Smith's 18th-century work on the *Theory of Moral Sentiments* ([1790] 2009) shows with his psychological device of the 'impartial spectator' how the emotional aspects of our morality can be included in practical reasoning.

There is a legal context to health care, and the moral dilemmas which arise involve legal and the moral aspects which are closely linked. We have seen classic legal cases that show the complexity of moral aspects of the argument and also the difficulties which exist when we try to enshrine a moral principle in law. In this connection MacCormick asks:

> Does a moral assessment of the facts of the matter simply replicate the legal, or is a different approach possible and appropriate? ... legal reasoning is a different instance of practical reasoning from moral reasoning. Neither is a mere subset of the other, though there are important analogies and similarities between them. (2008:192)

We saw in the landmark case of negligence in the 'snail in the bottle' case that the moral argument seemed straightforward and was easily demonstrated, but the legal case was harder to make. Whereas in the case of the Maltese conjoined twins, the legal position was clear, however there remained moral discomfiture after the judgement.

Ethics and Teamwork

Teamwork is much more talked about than brought off successfully. The basis of good teamwork is open communication and good record-keeping and sharing. We must take as a given that mutual respect for different team members and disciplines prevails. A collaborative, teamwork approach to health care ethics sits well with the working practices and management style of advanced health service organisations. One of the mainstays of such a service is what is known as 'clinical governance'; this is variously defined, but a succinct and accurate definition is 'corporate accountability for clinical performance'.[1] Clinical governance is an organisational system for delivering quality care; it might also show itself to be a good model for handling the moral aspects of care and for handling the ethical questions that arise in practice.

As we have said, the incorporation of the moral aspect of care into health service delivery is a practical matter and comes down to the point made earlier and rendered as the slogan 'If you can do teamwork, you can do ethics'. The 'posh' version of this could be expressed in terms of *clinical governance* and its ethical equivalent, which

---

[1]Galbraith, S. Management Executive Letter (MEL) 'Clinical governance', 1998. Scottish Executive Health Department.

for the purposes of explanation we might call *ethical governance*. Teamwork is the organisational model for delivering health care, and collaborative ethical discussion takes place on a multi-professional team basis. The organisation and structure within which these activities take place is important, as it sets the context and the habit (remember Aristotle) of the practice. The result is that the members of the team are accustomed to working together, holding ward rounds, case meetings and so on to agree plans for care and clinical management.

Ethical concerns are part of this set-up and need to have the same structures and practices in place. We can think of it in terms of a pairing of *clinical governance*, that being the organisation's means of achieving effective, quality health care, with *ethical governance*, the means of ensuring that practice also meets ethical standards. If we think of ethics and teamwork in partnership, then the benefits should be twofold. Engaging in ethical discussion of specific cases allows team members to understand one another. And if teamwork is the organisational structure within which different professions work and understand, then this everyday organisational fact paves the way for routinely including a consideration of the moral aspects of health care.

Multi-professional Ethical Discussion

So far I have largely avoided using the label 'nursing ethics', preferring to regard ethics for nursing practice as part of a collaborative approach to health care ethics. I have argued elsewhere for a collaborative approach to health care ethics, which involved a retreat from the idea of 'nursing ethics', largely because the original model of medical ethics with nursing ethics sitting alongside seemed to propel nursing into the position of some kind of counterweight or corrective to medical practice and ethics. The argument went like this:

> It would be a better idea to promote health care ethics, rather than continuing with the present parallel existence of medical ethics and nursing ethics literatures and debates. This formulation would put the patient in the centre and emphasise the importance of inter-disciplinary teamwork in the health care system. (Melia, 2004: 6)

However, the label 'nursing ethics' has taken firm root in the literature of the discipline and remains an important basis for nursing practice, and so to seek to re-badge nursing ethics, and for that matter medical ethics, as a part of health care ethics is probably a fool's errand. It is perhaps more important that health care professionals understand one another's ethical concerns and positions on specific matters.[2]

Nursing ethics has a tendency to be somewhat adversarial, and this, I think, has at times made collaborative ethics difficult. This tendency is most clearly seen in the

---

[2]A good example is the joint statement on CPR and a unified approach to clinical judgement (DNAR, 2007).

writings on 'nurse as the patient's advocate', where the position adopted is that the nurse is well placed to be the patient's advocate.

The main problem is that advocacy has adversarial connotations. An adversarial relationship between the two professions is not helping the cause of patient autonomy, nor is it especially collegial. A combination of the nurse as advocate and the increasing appearance of the patient as litigant could threaten the future of collaborative ethics.

However all that may be, there is something to be said for the existence of nursing ethics, qua nursing ethics from which nursing's view can develop as one view among others to be woven into the collaborative ethical discussion. The result is a working pattern of a collaborative multi-disciplinary health care team, which can explore ethical aspects of care as a team in much the same way as the team plans and undertakes patient care.

Multi-disciplinary anything is only as good as the contributions of the constituent disciplines. In the case of health care ethics the views of the various disciplines in health care feed into collaborative ethics, and these views may provide a different perspective, may at times be a corrective, or result in a useful amendment to the final decision. MacCormick noted that 'moral opinions are relevant to law, or at least to law reform' (2008: 181). In a similar way, nursing ethics can provide a useful contribution to collaborative ethical debate in a way that is different from erstwhile nursing ethics, reacting, as it were, against medical ethics. This is not a weak position for nursing to adopt, rather it is a constructive role and a means of weaving nursing's ideas into ethical debate and influencing collaborative ethics in health care practice.

To Conclude

The safe practice of professionals and the good workings of organised health care ultimately come down to trust. Trust is a central ethical concept in all that we have discussed and it figures clearly among the essential virtues for nurses and members of the other health care professions. The law can provide regulatory systems and enshrine some of the morally desirable practices in law. This, as we have seen, is not always as easily achieved as might be supposed.

All of this brings us back to the idea of trust. Onora O'Neill, in the opening of her first lecture in her 2002 Reith Lectures[3] on the BBC, said:

> Each of us and every profession and every institution needs trust. We need it because we have to be able to rely on others acting as they say they will, and because we need others to accept that we will act as we say we will. (2002: 4)

---

[3]The BBC Reith Lectures 2002, *A Question of Trust*.

This seems to be a fitting thought on which end to this book. The challenge[4] is how to arrive at this position of trust without imposing such regulated uniformity that the virtues with which the professions traditionally were imbued are lost in a stultifying storm of regulation, which would bring its own difficulties and not advance the cause of ethics for nursing and health care practice.

---

[4]The challenge is a specific one for the implementation of the Francis Report (2013) following the Mid Staffordshire Inquiry. Keogh (2013) has perhaps recognised this in his 'achievable ambitions' approach to the recommendations of the Francis Report.

Further Reading and Web Resources

Law and Ethics

Kuhse, H. and Singer, P. (eds) (2009) *Companion to Bioethics*. Chichester: Wiley-Blackwell.
Dimond, B. (2011) *Legal Aspects of Nursing* (6th edn). Harlow: Pearson.
Hope, T., Savulescu, J. and Hendrick, J. (2008) *Medical Ethics and Law: The Core Curriculum* (2nd edn). London: Churchill Livingstone Elsevier.
Huxtable, R. (2012) *Law, Ethics and Compromise at the Limits of Life: To Treat or Not to Treat?* London: Routledge.
Mason, J.K. and Laurie, G.T. (2011) *Mason and McCall Smith's Law and Medical Ethics* (8th edn). Oxford: Oxford University Press.

Sociology

Useful discussions of sociology as applied to health care and the health care professions.
Clarke, A. (2010) *The Sociology of Healthcare* (2nd edn). Harlow: Pearson.
Ham, C. (2009) *Health Policy in Britain*. Basingstoke: Palgrave Macmillan.
Nettleton, S. (2013) *The Sociology of Health and Illness*. London: Wiley.
Scambler, G. (ed.) (2008) *Sociology as Applied to Medicine* (6th edn). London: Saunders.

Websites

British Medical Association: http://bma.org.uk/
General Medical Council: www.gmc-uk.org/
International Council of Nursing: www.icn.ch/about-icn/
National Research Ethics Service, with links to sites concerned with ethics and research: www.nres.nhs.uk/
Nursing and Midwifery Council: www.nmc-uk.org/
The Health Foundation, an independent charity working to improve the quality of health care in the UK: www.health.org.uk/

Bibliography

Allen, D. (2001) *The Changing Shape of Nursing Practice*. London: Routledge.

Atkinson, P. (1995) *Medical Talk and Medical Work: The Liturgy of the Clinic*. London: SAGE.

Beauchamp, T.M. and Childress J.C. (2001) *Principles of Biomedical Ethics* (5th edn). Oxford: Oxford University Press.

Benedictus, D. and Clark, B. (1982) *Whose Life is it Anyway?* London: Sphere.

Boyd, K.M. (1999) 'Advance directives: the ethical implications', *Scottish Journal of Healthcare Chaplaincy*, 2: 3–7.

Boyd, K.M. (2002) 'Editorial: the law, death and medical ethics: Mrs Pretty and Ms B', *Journal of Medical Ethics*, 28(4): 211–12.

Bristol Royal Infirmary Inquiry (2001) *Learning from Bristol: The Report of the Public Inquiry into Children's Heart Surgery at BRI 1984–1995* (The Kennedy Report). Cmnd Paper CM5207. Norwich: Stationery Office. Available at: www.bristol-inquiry.org.uk.

British Medical Association (2009) *Medical Ethics Today* (2nd edn). London: BMJ Publishing Group.

Campbell, A. (2003) *NICE or Nasty? Threats to Justice from an Emphasis on Effectiveness*. London: Nuffield Trust.

Campbell, A.V. (1984) *Moral Dilemmas in Medicine* (3rd edn). Edinburgh: Churchill Livingstone.

Campbell, A.V., Gillett, G. and Jones, G. (2005) *Medical Ethics* (4th edn). Oxford: Oxford University Press.

Clarke, A. (2010) *The Sociology of Healthcare* (2nd edn). Harlow: Pearson.

Clothier Report (1994) *The Allitt Inquiry: An Independent Inquiry Relating to the Deaths and Injuries on the Children's Ward at Grantham and Kesteven General Hospital During the Period February to April 1991*. London: HMSO.

Department of Health (DH) (2000) *The NHS Plan: A Plan for Investment, a Plan for Reform*. London: Stationery Office.

Dimond, B. (2011) *Legal Aspects of Nursing* (6th edn). Harlow: Pearson.

DNAR (2007) *Decisions Relating to Cardiopulmonary Resuscitation: A Joint Statement*. London: British Medical Association, the Resuscitation Council (UK) and the Royal College of Nursing.

Francis, R. (2013) *Independent Inquiry into Care Provided by Mid Staffordshire NHS Foundation Trust, January 2005–March 2009*. London: Stationery Office.

Frankena, W.K. (1973) *Ethics* (2nd edn). Englewood Cliffs, NJ: Prentice Hall.

Freidson, E. (1970) *Profession of Medicine*. New York: Dodd Mead.

Freidson, E. (2001) *Professionalism the Third Logic*. Cambridge: Polity Press.

Giddens, A. (1997) *Sociology* (3rd edn). Cambridge: Polity Press.

Gilligan, C. (1982) *In a Different Voice: Psychological Theory and Women's Development*. Cambridge, MA: Harvard University Press.

Gillon, R. (1994) 'The four principles revisited: a reappraisal', in R. Gillon and A. Lloyd (eds), *Principles of Health Care Ethics*. Chichester: Wiley.

Gillon, R. and Lloyd, A. (eds) (1994) *Principles of Health Care Ethics*. Chichester: Wiley.

Ham, C. (2009) *Health Policy in Britain*. Basingstoke: Palgrave Macmillan.

Henderson, V. (1964) *The Nature of Nursing*. London: Collier Macmillan.

Hope, T., Savulescu, J. and Hendrick, J. (2008) *Medical Ethics and Law: The Core Curriculum* (2nd edn). London: Churchill Livingstone Elsevier.

Hume, D. (1739) *A Treatise of Human Nature: Being an Attempt to Introduce the Experimental Method of Reasoning into Moral Subjects*.

Hume, D. ([1739] 1978) *A Treatise of Human Nature* (L. A. Selby-Bigge and P. H. Nidditch, eds). Oxford: Clarendon Press.

Hume, D. ([1777] 1978) *A Treatise of Human Nature* (2nd edn, L.A. Selby-Bigge and P.H. Nidditch, eds). Oxford: Clarendon Press.

Hume, D. ([1777] 1902) *Enquiries Concerning the Human Understanding: And Concerning the Principles of Morals* (L.A. Selby-Bigge, ed.). Oxford: Clarendon Press.

Huxtable, R. (2012) *Law, Ethics and Compromise at the Limits of Life: To Treat or Not to Treat?* London: Routledge.

Jonsen, A. and Toulmin, S. (1988) *The Abuse of Casuistry: A History of Moral Reasoning*. Berkeley: University of California Press.

Kant, I. ([1785] 1953) *Groundwork of the Metaphysic of Morals* (trans. H. Paton). London: Hutchinson.

Kant, I. ([1787] 1973) *Critique of Practical Reason* (trans. L.W. Beck). Indianapolis, IN: Bobbs-Merrill.

Kohlberg, L. (1981) The Philosophy of Moral Development. San Francisco: Harper and Row.

Kuhse, H. and Singer, P. (eds) (2009) *Companion to Bioethics*. Chichester: Wiley-Blackwell.

Larrabee, M.J. (ed.) (1993) *An Ethic of Care: Feminist and Interdisciplinary Perspectives*. New York: Routledge.

Local Government Association, NHS Confederation, Age UK (2012) *Delivering Dignity: Securing Dignity in Care for Older People in Hospitals and Care*. Available at: www.nhsconfed.org/Publications/reports/Pages/Delivering-Dignity.aspx.

Lyon, D. (1965) *The Forms and Limits of Utilitarianism*. Oxford: Oxford University Press.

MacCormick, N. (2008) *Practical Reason in Law and Morality*. Oxford: Oxford University Press.

MacQueen, H.L. (1999) *Studying Scots Law* (2nd edn). Edinburgh: Butterworth.

Mason, J.K. and Laurie, G.T. (2011) *Mason and McCall Smith's Law and Medical Ethics* (8th edn). Oxford: Oxford University Press.

Mayo, B. (1986) *The Philosophy of Right and Wrong*. London: Routledge and Kegan Paul.

McLean, S. (2010) *Autonomy, Consent and the Law*. London: Routledge Cavendish.

Melia, K.M. (1987) *Learning and Working: The Occupational Socialization of Nurses*. London: Tavistock.

Melia, K.M. (2004) *Health Care Ethics: Lessons from Intensive Care*. London: SAGE.

Melia, K.M. (2011) 'About decision making at the end of life: case commentary', *Asian Bioethics Review*, 3(2): 145–9.

Mill, J.S. ([1863] 1962) 'Utilitarianism', in J.S. Mill (1962) *Utilitarianism, On Liberty, Essay on Bentham Together with Selected Writings of Jeremy Bentham and John Austin*. (M. Warnock, ed.). London: Fontana.

Nettleton, S. (2013) *The Sociology of Health and Illness*. London: Wiley.

Nursing and Midwifery Council (2004) *NMC Guidance: Requirements for Evidence of Good Health and Good Character*. London: Nursing and Midwifery Council.

Nursing and Midwifery Council (2008) *NMC Code of Professional Conduct: Standards for Performance, Conduct and Ethics*. London: Nursing and Midwifery Council.

Nursing and Midwifery Council (2011) *Guidance on Professional Conduct for Nursing and Midwifery Students* (3rd edn). London: Nursing and Midwifery Council.

O'Neill, O. (1993) 'Kantian ethics', in P. Singer (ed.), *A Companion to Ethics*. Oxford: Blackwell, pp. 175–85.

O'Neill, O. (2002) *A Question of Trust: The BBC Reith Lectures 2002*. Cambridge: Cambridge University Press.

Parliamentary and Health Service Ombudsman (2011) *Care and Compassion?* Available at: www.ombudsman.org.uk/care-and-compassion.

Priest, S. (1990) *The British Empiricists*. London: Penguin.

Prime Minister's Commission on the Future of Nursing and Midwifery in England (2010) *Front Line Care*. London: Stationery Office. Available at: http://cnm.independent.gov.uk.

Rietjens, J.A.C., van der Maas, P.J., Onwuteaka-Philipsen, B.J., van Delden, J.J.M. and van der Heide, A. (2009) 'Two decades of research on euthanasia from the Netherlands. What have we learnt and what questions remain', *Bioethical Inquiry*, 6: 271–83 .

Royal College of Nursing (2010) *Guidance on Safe Nurse Staffing Levels in the UK*. Publication code: 003 860. London: Royal College of Nursing. Available at www.rcn.org.uk (accessed 3 March 2012).

Royal College of Nursing (2012) *Mandatory Staffing Levels: Policy Briefing*. London: Royal College of Nursing.

Scambler, G. (ed.) (2008) *Sociology as Applied to Medicine* (6th edn). London: Saunders.

Singer, P. (1993) *Practical Ethics* (2nd edn). Cambridge: Cambridge University Press.

Singer, P. (ed.) (1994) *Ethics* (2nd edn). Oxford: Oxford University Press.

Singer, P. (2002) 'Ms B and Diane Pretty: a commentary', *Journal of Medical Ethics*, 28(4): 234–5.

Smart, J.J.C. and Williams, B. (1973) *Utilitarianism: For and Against*. Cambridge: Cambridge University Press.

Smith, A. ([1776] 1999) *The Wealth of Nations: Books I–III*. London: Penguin Classics.

Smith, A. ([1790] 2009) *The Theory of Moral Sentiments* (6th edn, edited with notes by R.P. Hanley). London: Penguin.

Starkey, J. (2010) 'Blood, guts and a chance of life', *The Times*, 20 November.

Syal, R. (2013) 'Second whistleblower claims NHS chief ignored hospital warnings', *The Guardian*, 15 February.

Thomson J.A.K. (1976) *The Ethics of Aristotle – The Nicomachean Ethics*. Harmondsworth: Penguin (many other translations are available).

Toulmin, S. (1981) The 'tyranny of principles', *Hastings Center Report*, 11: 31–9.

Zussman, R. (1992) *Intensive Care: Medical Ethics and the Medical Profession*. Chicago, IL: University of Chicago Press.

Index